A GUIDE FOR
HELPING THE CHILD
WITH SPINA BIFIDA

A GUIDE FOR HELPING THE CHILD WITH SPINA BIFIDA

Edited by

GARY J. MYERS, M.D.

*Associate Professor of Pediatrics
and Director
Center for Developmental and Learning Disorders
University of Alabama
Birmingham, Alabama*

SHARON BIDWELL CERONE, R.N., M.S.N.

*Nurse Clinician (Pediatrics)
Assistant Professor of Nursing and Pediatrics
University of Rochester
Rochester, New York*

ARDIS L. OLSON, M.D.

*Clinical Assistant Professor
Department of Pediatrics
Children's Hospital at Stanford
Stanford University Medical Center
Palo, Alto, California*

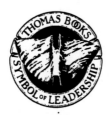

CHARLES C THOMAS • PUBLISHER
Springfield • Illinois • U.S.A.

Published and Distributed Throughout the World by

CHARLES C THOMAS • PUBLISHER

Bannerstone House

301-327 East Lawrence Avenue, Springfield, Illinois, U.S.A.

© *1981, by* CHARLES C THOMAS • PUBLISHER

ISBN 0-398-04113-X

Library of Congress Catalog Card Number: 80-17953

With THOMAS BOOKS *careful attention is given to all details of
manufacturing and design. It is the Publisher's desire to present books that
are satisfactory as to their physical qualities and artistic possibilities and
appropriate for their particular use.* THOMAS BOOKS *will be true to those
laws of quality that assure a good name and good will.*

Printed in the United States of America
V-R-1

Library of Congress Cataloging in Publication Data

Main entry under title:
 A Guide for helping the child with spina bifida.
 Includes index.
 1. Spina bibida. I. Myers, Gary J.
II. Cerone, Sharon Bidwell. III. Olson, Ardis L.
[DNLM: 1. Spina bifida--Popular works. WE730
G946]
RJ496.S74G84   617'.375   80-17953
ISBN 0-398-04113-X

CONTRIBUTORS

Steven M. Adair, D.D.S., M.S.
Assistant Chairman, Department of Pedodontics, Eastman Dental Center; Assistant Professor of Clinical Dentistry, University of Rochester School of Medicine and Dentistry.

Hilda Banfield
Parent.

Judy Brede
Young adult with spina bifida.

Marilyn R. Brown, M.D.
Associate Professor of Pediatrics (Gastroenterology)
Assistant Professor of Medicine, Birth Defects Center, University of Rochester.

Mary Ann Campbell, R.N., M.S.
Nurse Clinician (Pediatrics, Gastroenterology)
Instructor in Nursing, Birth Defects Center, University of Rochester.

Sharon Bidwell Cerone, R.N., M.S.N.
Nurse Clinician (Pediatrics),
Assistant Professor of Nursing and Pediatrics, University of Rochester, Formerly, Nurse Clinician and Coordinator, Birth Defects Center.

Margaret T. Colgan, M.D.
Associate Professor of Pediatrics,
Director of Ambulatory Pediatrics and The Birth Defects Center, University of Rochester.

Jeanette Felix, Ph.D.
Assistant Professor of Pediatrics, Johns Hopkins University.

Carey Gunther
Young adult with spina bifida.

Martha Gram, B.S., R.P.T.
Physical Therapist, Birth Defects Center, University of Rochester Medical Center.

Anne and Robert Griswold
Parents.

P. William Haake, M.D.
Clinical Associate Professor of Surgery (Orthopaedics), Birth Defects Center, University of Rochester and Genesee Hospital.

Ursula Hage, R.N., B.S.
Liaison Nurse, Monroe County Department of Public Health Nursing and Birth Defects Center, University of Rochester.

Catherine E. Hannon, M.S.S.A., A.C.S.W.
Senior Social Worker, Regional Early Childhood Direction Center, Formerly, Birth Defects Center, University of Rochester.

Kenneth V. Jackman, M.D.
Assistant Professor of Surgery (Orthopaedics) and Pediatrics, Birth Defects Center, University of Rochester Medical Center.

Laverne and David Judge
Parents.

Harold A. Kanthor, M.D.
Clinical Assistant Professor of Pediatrics, University of Rochester, Joseph Wilson Health Center, Rochester, New York.

Harriet J. Kitzman, R.N., M.S.
Doctoral student in nursing, formerly, Chief of Pediatric Nursing, Associate Professor of Nursing and Pediatrics, University of Rochester.

Calvin Lauder, M.A.
Coordinator of Student Educational Services, City School District, Rochester, New York.

Jane Wheeler Legg, B.S.
Family Counselor, formerly, Birth Defects Center, University of Rochester.

Barbara Leonard
Illustrator of "Sue Stone's Guitar Recital."

Mira L. Lessick, R.N., M.S.
Doctoral student in Nursing, formerly, Nurse Clinician (Pediatrics, Genetics), Assistant Professor of Nursing, University of Rochester.

Clinton Lillibridge, M.D.
Pediatrician and Gastroenterologist, Rochester, New York.

Gwendolyn Marshman, R.N.
Nurse Clinician (Orthopaedics), University of Rochester.

Joseph V. McDonald, M.D.
Professor and Chairman of Surgery (Neurosurgery), University of Rochester.

Eileen and John Moreland
Parents.

Joan Alexander Moxley
Illustrator of Text.

Gary J. Myers, M.D.
Associate Professor of Pediatrics and Director, Center for Developmental and Learning Disorders, University of Alabama in Birmingham. Formerly, Director, Birth Defects Center, University of Rochester.

Robert Nitschke
Orthotist and Prosthetist, Rochester Orthopaedic Laboratory and Birth Defects Center, University of Rochester.

Shige-Hisa Okawara, M.D.
Associate Professor of Surgery (Neurosurgery), Birth Defects Center, University of Rochester.

Ardis L. Olson, M.D.
Clinical Assistant Professor, Department of Pediatrics, Children's Hospital at Stanford, Stanford University Medical Center.

Helen R. Patterson
Field Consultant, National Action for Foster Children, formerly, Executive Director, Child Health Advisory Group, Department of Pediatrics, Parents and Financial Coordinator, Birth Defects Center, University of Rochester.

Franklin V. Peale, M.D.
Clinical Assistant Professor of Surgery (Orthopaedics) Birth Defects Center, University of Rochester and Genesee Hospital.

Marjorie C. Pfaudler, R.N., M.A.
Nurse Clinician (Adult Rehabilitation), Associate Professor of Nursing and Preventive Medicine and Community Health, University of Rochester.

Ronald Rabinowitz, M.D.
Assistant Professor of Surgery (Urology) and Pediatrics, Birth Defects Center, University of Rochester Medical Center and Rochester General Hospital.

Nancy Rice
Chief Social Worker (Pediatrics), Instructor in Health Services and Pediatrics, University of Rochester.

Olle Jane Z. Sahler, M.D.
Assistant Professor of Pediatrics and Psychiatry, University of Rochester.

Mary Jane Schneider, B.S., E.T.
Enterostomal Therapist in Private Practice, formerly, Birth Defects Center, University of Rochester.

Rune J. Simeonsson, Ph.D.
Assistant Professor of Pediatrics, Psychiatry and Psychology, University of Rochester.

Albert C. Snell, M.D.
Professor of Opthalmology (Emeritus), University of Rochester.

Winifred C. Stebbins, Ed.M.
Educational Specialist, Coordinator, School Health Program, Instructor in Pediatrics, University of Rochester.

Karen and Edward Steitler
Parents.

Odd Bjarne Sveen, Ph.D., D.D.S.
Chairman, Department of Pedodontics, Eastman Dental Center, Associate Professor of Clinical Dentistry, Dental Research, and Pediatrics, Birth Defects Center and Eastman Dental Center, University of Rochester.

Phillip L. Townes, M.D.
Professor of Pediatrics, University of Massachusetts.

Donna and Louis Wilkes
Parents.

FOREWORD

THIS volume provides an account of the problems confronting parents and their children with Spina Bifida. It is written for parents, health professionals and educators who are concerned with any aspect of care for children with Spina Bifida.

All parents of children born with Spina Bifida and all professionals who work on behalf of these children face continuing educational problems, which require constant interchange among and between parents and professionals who are constantly looking for new and better methods of maximizing the potential of children with Spina Bifida.

This volume provides an easily understandable, comprehensive, and authoritative account of the variety of problems which are present in the newborn, the developmental aspects of the multiple facets of the defect, and the distinctive role which a variety of specialists and health professionals play in providing the essential care required by these children. It is not designed to be placed in the hands of a new parent who, for the first time, is asking: "What is this birth defect?" and "What problems will confront my child?" The comprehensive treatment of the subject provides too much information for such parents. This book is most suitable for individuals with some understanding, who want to learn more about Spina Bifida in general or some specific aspect.

This useful work will successfully fill an unmet need of all who are concerned with the habilitation of children with Spina Bifida and, in addition to factual information about the birth defect, will clearly indicate to parents the type of interdisciplinary care which can most effectively provide those services.

Chester A. Swinyard, M.D., Ph.D.
Visiting Professor Emeritus of Surgery
(Rehabilitation Medicine)
Children's Hospital at Stanford

ACKNOWLEDGMENTS

THE idea of writing a book to guide parents and others in helping children with spina bifida originated during a conference on spina bifida. When we presented the concept to our colleagues in The Birth Defects Center at Strong Memorial Hospital, Rochester, New York, they were unanimous in enthusiastically supporting the idea. We then contacted families and many other individuals who had personal experience with spina bifida, and most eagerly concurred and agreed to help. These individuals either contributed to this book or assisted us in preparing it. Each contributor shared his or her personal views and expertise, and the Editors then organized and revised the material so the book would be more cohesive and could be easily read and understood.

The Birth Defects Center was originally founded by the National Foundation-March of Dimes. Later, the local chapter of that organization continued to actively support the Center after the grant expired. For several years now, the Easter Seal Society has been instrumental in seeing that the work of the Center continues. Both the Department of Pediatrics in the School of Medicine and Dentistry, and the School of Nursing of the University of Rochester have supported the Center continuously since its inception. We wish to express our sincere thanks to all these groups. Without the support of The Birth Defects Center and its personnel, this book would not have been possible.

The families and children with whom we worked in The Birth Defects Center deserve special recognition for their patience, understanding, and cooperation. They provided the inspiration which sustained us through the difficulties of completing such a book. Many of them also contributed their experiences, time, ideas, and advice to the text. They even provided the photographic subjects to illustrate the manuscipt. We are sincerely grateful to the adults and children with spina bifida, their brothers and sisters, parents, and relatives for all their assistance.

A special acknowledgment is due to Mrs. Sondra Myers, Mrs. Patty Ford, and Mrs. Carol Cleveland for their secretarial and editorial assistance. Dr. Sarah Davis and Dr. Richard Admussen were kind enough to review and comment upon the manuscript. Without the combined talents and efforts of all these individuals, this manuscript might still be incomplete.

Gary J. Myers
Sharon Bidwell Cerone
Ardis L. Olson

INTRODUCTION

SPINA BIFIDA (pronounced spy-na-by-fida) is a common birth defect. Spina refers to the backbone or spine, while bifida means divided into two parts. In this birth defect a part of the spine, which normally surrounds and protects the spinal cord or nervous tissue, fails to form a complete ring and the parts remain separated. Spina bifida is a general term, and there are several specific types. Each type carries a different outlook. Some individuals with the "hidden form" of spina bifida may lead a normal life and never be aware of the defect. However, other types of spina bifida are more serious, and it is the nonfatal but serious types that this book focuses upon. About 3000 infants are born in the United States each year with such defects, and throughout the world there are many times this number.

Although many recent medical advances have helped these children, we feel the family continues to play the central and largest role in helping the child. Since families, and especially parents, are so important for the child with spina bifida, we decided to write this book to help you. Many excellent books on the child with spina bifida are already in print, but they are primarily directed to professionals. We have attempted to provide information on a level that parents can understand. Our overall philosophy has been to provide a *positive* approach tempered by *realism*. We feel the difference between successful and unsuccessful parenting depends primarily on whether you believe that you can accomplish the task of rearing a special child.

We believe parents are anxious to learn how to provide better care for their loved one with spina bifida. The recent consumer self-help movement has reinforced our opinion that people want to understand more fully both how and why the care should be provided. Understanding your child's defect should reduce the anxiety created by not knowing, and make you more effective in your child's care. We hope that parents who are more understanding, knowledgeable, and self-assured will also be more optimistic. Such a positive attitude toward your child can be a major factor in helping him.

You will note that we chose the term "disabled" over "handicapped." The increasingly vocal disabled minority in our society has correctly made a distinction between these terms. "Disabled" is a state over which one has no control. Either a birth defect or an accident

xiii

may prevent one from doing certain tasks because a body part is missing or not functioning properly. A "handicapped" person, however, can be prevented from accomplishing tasks for many reasons. A poor attitude in any person is a serious handicap. Preventing the disabled from being handicapped is a central focus of this book.

We have chosen to refer to both children and professionals as "he." Although spina bifida affects as many girls as boys and many health care givers and educators are female, we felt a consistent writing style was important.

This book comes from the experiences the authors have had and those that numerous families have shared with us. It grew out of a working relationship between numerous health professionals and families and children affected by spina bifida. In our Birth Defects Center, a considerable amount of staff time was spent on basic education of families about spina bifida. We felt that if parents had a source of information where they could begin to understand the problems, then the Center could be a second level of inquiry and there would be more time for meaningful discussion. We have tried to concentrate on practical information that parents might find useful.

Parents and professionals usually gain their knowledge about children with spina bifida from different sources. Families are often very familiar with the practical aspects of their child's care, while health professionals are more knowledgeable and concerned with the medical aspects. Consequently, some professionals may not adequately appreciate a family's practical skills and life experiences, or families may lose sight of the professional's medical ability. This can result in communication problems between the family and the health professionals. Mutual understanding and open discussion of these issues is one key to obtaining the best care for your child.

We set out to produce a reference book that families could have available and refer to as questions arose. Our plan was to be as comprehensive as possible in order to help those families where the problem does arise. Both sides of certain controversial issues, and even some outmoded ideas and techniques, have been included for completeness. However, children with spina bifida vary greatly, and parts of the text may not apply now or at any future time to your child or your family. Most children with spina bifida have only some of the problems discussed. Contents, Glossary, and a cross-referenced Index, hopefully, should help you find the information you are seeking. The *Guide* may be helpful either before or after medical visits, when discussion of a problem is anticipated, or an explanation was not fully understood. It was not designed to be read from cover to cover, and we hope each chapter or section can be understood individually. When you become interested in a topic, simply turn to the Index or to the chapter covering that subject.

The text has been organized into four major sections. The first discusses general issues, the second specific medical problems, the third presents the views of families who have had personal contact with spina bifida, and the fourth is a children's story about a young girl with spina bifida. It was difficult to decide where some topics belong, but we have tried to keep special medical services in the second section. The general issues have been further divided according to the child's development. We chose to discuss infancy (birth through one year), childhood (one year to the teens), and the teenage years separately. Each developmental period includes the major events that usually occur during that time. Most medical problems are not confined to developmental stages and are not divided in this manner. The third section on family views presents a cross-section of individuals of varying sexes, races, and ages, including adults.

It is important to recognize that each child is an individual both in personality and in the exact nature and extent of the medical problems. Spina bifida is a general term, and children who look very similar often have very different medical and social needs. Although this *Guide* can help you to understand your child with spina bifida better, applying this knowledge to an individual child is more complex. Your child's own health care providers should understand his special needs better than anyone else and be able to assist you in providing the best possible care. You should feel free to discuss any of your concerns with them. Children with spina bifida have several diverse problems. Consequently, a variety of health· specialists may need to help with your child's care. When they are available, we feel, a group of specialists working as a team offers many advantages.

We hope you will find this *Guide* useful and that both you and your special child will benefit from what you learn. We believe that children with spina bifida can develop into happy, independent, and contributing members of our society. We also feel that knowledgeable and understanding parents are the key to achieving this goal.

CONTENTS

Section I
An Overview of the Child and the Family

Chapter

Section II
Understanding Your Child's Body Functions

xvii

A GUIDE FOR
HELPING THE CHILD
WITH SPINA BIFIDA

Section I

An Overview of the Child and the Family

CHAPTER 1

EVALUATING THE BABY
AND MAKING DECISIONS

The Evaluation

WHEN a child is born with spina bifida, he needs and deserves a thorough evaluation by a medical team. Whether this team is multidisciplinary (consists of many specialists) or is only your family doctor and a nurse, they will carefully consider each of the aspects which follow. Each of these can be assessed in a newborn, and every aspect of the evaluation will provide information which will help the health professionals gain a broad view of your child's disability.

No matter what problem may exist, your baby will need a thorough general physical examination. This is especially important since any infant with one congenital defect is more likely to have a second defect; and those that involve internal organs such as the heart, lungs or intestinal tract, may not be readily apparent. When no other defects are present, this is an important positive factor for your baby. If other defects are present, they must be considered in the overall picture.

The Open Spine

The back and the open spine (spina bifida) need careful examination. Important aspects are: (a) the size of the defect, (b) how many vertebrae are open or divided, (c) whether the opening is in the high, mid or lower part of the back, (d) whether the opening is covered with skin or with thin membranes, and (e) whether there is spinal fluid leaking from the opening.

When the area of open spine is very large or high on the back, it is more serious. However, leakage of spinal fluid is *the* most serious problem since infection can occur more readily.

Very large skin defects may be difficult to close surgically. In this case, skin grafts may be needed. Early surgical closure within the first few days is usually desirable, but sometimes the difficulty in deciding about the extent of the defect, the overall disability, or the approach to treatment will slow this down. If the defect is not surgically closed, skin will grow in from the sides and cover the defect. This sometimes makes later surgical closure easier.

5

The Head

Children with spina bifida frequently have hydrocephalus or excess fluid within the head. This may be present at birth or develop within the first few days or weeks of life. In infants, the bones of the skull are not joined together like they are in older children and adults. Therefore, as the volume of fluid within the brain increases, the head grows. It is fortunate the skull bones can separate, since the increased pressure from extra spinal fluid does not produce damage to the nervous tissue as quickly when this occurs. It may be necessary to measure the head size for several days, weeks or months to be certain whether surgery to relieve the pressure (shunt) is needed. If an operation to relieve the fluid and pressure through shunting can be avoided, it will reduce the chances for the long-term problems associated with the shunt itself. Sometimes a shunt is needed early and some doctors prefer to do the shunt before they operate to close the defect on the back. They feel that reducing the pressure around the nervous tissue helps the back to heal better. Although hydrocephalus seems to be present in most infants with spina bifida, some do not develop enough hydrocephalus to require an operation to relieve the pressure.

The Paralysis

When the spine is open, there is usually damage to the nerves and spinal cord near the defect. When the opening is large enough that the skin does not cover it or there is a bulge on the back, the nervous system is usually more seriously affected.

The involvement of nerves and spinal cord differs greatly in each individual child. In some children, there will be paralysis of all the muscles below the back defect, but in others there may be only partial paralysis. This paralysis is permanent and usually does not change later. There is often a difference between the two legs in terms of movement and feeling. Any movement which occurs in the legs or any feeling which is present will be helpful to your child later, especially when he tries to be mobile. Sometimes there appears to be movement in the legs, especially when they are touched or handled. This type of movement may be a reflex and may never come under the child's voluntary control.

Urinary Control

A careful evaluation of bladder and kidney function is needed, since the nerves very low in the back control the bladder. These nerves are damaged to some extent in nearly all cases of spina bifida when there is a skin defect on the back. This can lead to several urinary problems, particularly susceptability to urine infections and difficulty in becoming toilet trained at a later age.

A bladder with a damaged nervous supply can lead to urine backing up (reflux) and cause enlarged kidneys (hydronephosis). Both of these problems can occur in infancy and should be diagnosed and treated early, since proper kidney function is essential for long-term survival. These problems usually respond well to treatment if they are recognized early.

The Orthopedic Evaluation

Although the open spine can be closed surgically, open vertebrae cannot be surgically put back together. A search by x-ray of the other spine bones must be made, since there may be other abnormalities at any point along the spine. These may affect later growth of the spine and result in curvature of the spine (scoliosis). Where the vertebrae are open in the defect, the abnormal bones may be bent forward and a bony lump may be present. This may need surgical correction at a later time.

In addition to the spine, each of the joints (hip, knee, ankle) in the leg needs careful assessment. At times, the paralysis, which was present when the baby was still in the uterus leads to joints that are frozen in one position. This is termed arthrogryposis. Because of varying degrees of leg muscle paralysis, the hips may not be properly in the socket or the feet may be clubbed or there may be other abnormalities. All of the problems with bones and joints require early treatment. If treatment is delayed for several weeks, then the problem may ultimately be harder to correct.

Making Important Decisions

Medical technology seems to have progressed more rapidly than society's thinking about the disabled (i.e. prejudices, attitudes) or the provision of humanitarian support services (i.e. schooling, financial aid). Although society has made major strides in recent years, a gap still exists and questions must be asked about what "quality of life" can certain children with severe forms of spina bifida achieve. If the quality will be poor, is it ethical to place a child and family in a situation requiring society's help when that support may be lacking? Can society really offer children with a very serious birth defect a fair chance of achieving an acceptable "quality of life." All families and health personnel struggle with this issue, but it is a greater problem when the infant has one of the very severe forms of spina bifida.

Following the initial evaluation, it will be necessary to decide about surgery on the open spine. A poorly covered opening, which may be leaking spinal fluid, is at risk for infection. Because this may present such an urgent problem, it is sometimes difficult to help parents understand the full meaning of their child's spina bifida at the time these decisions must be reached. It is unfortunate that families often have so little time to fully comprehend the seriousness of the defect prior to this operation, since closure of the back usually represents a commitment to a course of treatment which will profoundly affect the lives of the entire family for a very long time.

Should All Children with Spina Bifida Receive Extensive Medical Therapy?

Children with spina bifida vary a great deal in the seriousness of their defect. Some professionals and parents feel that all life deserves the best that medical technology is able to offer. Others feel the medical condition of some children may be so serious and the quality of life so poor that extraordinary measures to save or prolong life should not be used. Children with the more serious types of spina bifida, who do not receive extra medical care, often die in the first year of life. The smaller number who do not die within the first year may develop more severe problems than those with which they started.

Some professionals feel that the future can at least be partially predicted on the basis of past experiences. It is not possible for anyone to know which individuals will do well as opposed to those who will not. However, studies of large numbers of children with spina bifida have provided experience from which some general predictions can be made. When the following aspects were present at birth, studies have found that a better outcome (required fewer operations and hospitalizations) was likely:

(1) No hydrocephalus at birth
(2) Able to move some muscles below the waist
(3) No major abnormal curvatures of the spine
(4) No kidney damage
(5) No other birth defects
(6) No infection of the spinal fluid (meningitis, ventriculitis)

If the infant had any of these problems or was unable to move any muscles below the waist, the outlook was not as good. If the infant had two or more of the above, then the outlook became progressively worse.

How Can a Decision Be Reached?

It is best that decisions in such difficult situations involve health professionals who have an understanding of both your child and special knowledge about spina bifida. We feel that decisions made mutually by health professionals and parents are the best. This may not always be possible; therefore, it is important that the family have confidence in the health professionals caring for their child. Mutual trust, respect, and understanding between parents and professionals is the cornerstone for making the best decisions.

The Value of a Positive Attitude

Although the child with spina bifida has many positive attributes, attention usually focuses on the problems. The child may look perfectly normal, have a lusty cry, suck well and be very responsive; yet these normal findings may be overlooked or, at least, go unstressed. Families need to recognize and understand their child's abilities and potentials. This becomes essential when the decision is reached to proceed with extensive medical support.

The attitudes of families toward their child are often shaped in the first hours or days of the child's life. Early negative attitudes may take months or years to overcome. Unfortunately, health professionals sometimes neglect to provide the family with a balanced picture of both the negative aspects and the positive ones. Perhaps this is a side effect of the current legal climate which requires the health providers to completely describe the problems and any possible complication.

Parents should focus on what is right with their child, and professionals should help them do that. Families who accept their child, work with him, and are able to take a positive approach toward the disability seem best able to help their child. This positive attitude, in turn, helps the child to build a good image of himself; and this is a firm foundation for future success.

CHAPTER 2

FEELINGS OF PARENTS

FEELINGS OF PARENTS

Feelings After the Birth

WHEN a child with spina bifida is born into a family, it is usually an unexpected event. All parents hope for a perfect baby with no major problems. Your dreams during the pregnancy probably focused on such happy thoughts as how the baby would look and act and whether you would have a boy or girl. To be told that your child has spina bifida is surprising and upsetting news.

The birth of any baby is an emotional event for the parents, but it is a real crisis when the baby has a serious birth defect. Parents experience many kinds of quite strong feelings when this situation arises. They may feel shock, confusion, anger, frustration, and even disbelief and guilt. The intensity of these emotions may vary, but most parents experience similar feelings when they have a baby with spina bifida.

How Will You Manage?

How you responded to your infant's birth depended on your particular personality, your past experiences in life, and how you generally handle stress. Most parents experience moments during the early days of the infant's life when they are not sure they will be able to handle this new situation. Reviewing how parents often feel and how they react may help you to understand your own feelings after your baby was born.

Feeling Shocked by the News

Some parents feel shocked. They are usually confused about what is happening to them, frequently cry and simply feel helpless. They feel generally upset and do or say things that they ordinarily would not. A feeling of restlessness, anger, nervousness and an inability to eat, drink, or rest may also be present.

Disbelief

After the initial shock when the reality of the news takes hold, parents may begin to deny that their child has spina bifida. This sense

10

of disbelief is quite normal and common. The parents often hope that this situation will "just go away," or that some mistake has been made in the diagnosis. They may feel like they are in a dream and express feelings as "this can't really be happening to us." A sense of wanting to run away or hide may be present. This is an understandable response which most parents overcome fairly quickly.

Who Is to Blame?

As the seriousness of the baby's condition becomes clearer, parents often ask "Why us?" "What did we do to cause this problem?" A feeling of guilt and personal responsibility may begin to enter their thoughts. Feelings of being an inadequate father or mother may be present. Parents may ask, "Am I to blame?" "Am I bad or unworthy?"

In this state of emotional crisis, parents may blame each other or harbor secret resentment or fantasies that one or the other was responsible. This is a critical time for many families. Communication problems often arise when parents have intense feelings. It is more important than ever that parents share their feelings with each other during this crisis.

I Was Afraid the Baby Might Die

While parents are experiencing all these feelings, many also feel that something worse will happen to their child. This may even increase the feeling of grief and loss. They may have actually been told that it is uncertain whether their child will live or die. Because they fear their baby may die, parents may be reluctant to become close or attached to him. The closer one is to a loved one, the more it hurts when they are taken away. It is natural for all of us to try to protect ourselves from being hurt.

It is normal for parents to wonder if their child might not be better off dying now so as to spare further pain or suffering for all involved. This may produce increased guilt and shame. The honest expression of these feelings and realization that they are normal may help you to deal with these troubling thoughts.

What Happens to Parents' Feelings?

Whatever feelings you may experience, they will probably change as time passes. How they change varies with different individuals. Feelings that are pent up may turn inward and cause more sadness. If the feeling of helplessness and hopelessness is prolonged, it can become depression. Even if you handle such feelings in the best possible manner when your child is an infant, it is common to feel tinges of sadness about your child throughout life.

If such feelings become frustration, they may be turned outward and may be directed toward health professionals involved with your family at this difficult time. A parent may feel a particular person is responsible for the situation, for making it worse, or not providing the care they want and expect. Parents often vent this anger at those persons. Feelings of this nature can be best handled when you have free access to someone with whom you can talk. Professionals, like social workers, clergymen and psychologists can be most helpful at these times, since they are skilled in such matters and are not intimately involved in the medical care your child is receiving. Health professionals try to understand such hidden anger or sudden outbursts, but sometimes it is difficult.

How Do I Get to Know my Baby?

Most parents find that a period of great sadness or mourning needs to be experienced before their new baby with spina bifida is felt to be a part of the family. It is normal for parents to experience these feelings after birth, since they expected a healthy baby. This mourning process takes a long time to go away and may continue long after you feel you are coming to know your new child well. Touching, holding, feeding and all the other usual motherly and fatherly tasks will help you discover that the baby has his own personality and is really your baby. You may be surprised to find that the defect on the back is not as big a problem as you had imagined and that your child's responses to feeding and holding are just like any other infant's. The opportunity to see what is right with your baby is an important factor which will help you to develop a close and loving relationship. Your infant, like others, will be able to tell parents from strangers very early.

Reorganizing Your Life

As you begin to cope with some of these feelings and get to know your new child, a time of reorganizing your life occurs. Taking the baby home, beginning to see friends and relatives, and becoming involved with the community and other people will help. Meeting and talking with families who have personal experience helping a child with spina bifida can be especially reassuring. Returning to the daily routines of your life will contribute to generally feeling better about what lies ahead. You will feel more in control of your lives and have increased energy and ability to care for the new baby and the rest of the family.

Every child brings something special to his parents, and the child with spina bifida is no exception. As you become acquainted with your child, you will gradually begin to recognize and take pride in all the normal things he can do. You will also regain confidence in yourselves and your family. You will also realize that you are not alone and your child's day-by-day progress offers hope for his future and yours. Although the birth of a child with spina bifida is stressful to a family, most families are able to meet this challenge and handle it successfully. The rewards of this effort are very large. The child with spina bifida can bring something special into your lives, and this includes a great deal of happiness.

CHAPTER 3

CAUSES, RECURRENCE
AND PREVENTION

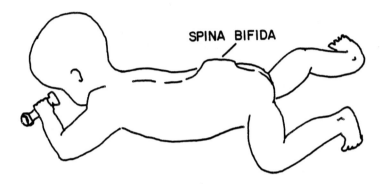

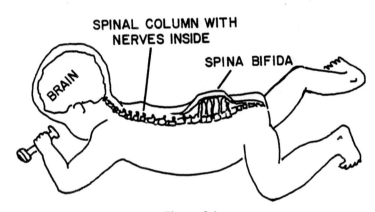

Figure 3-1.

CAUSES, RECURRENCE, AND PREVENTION

EXACTLY why spina bifida occurs is not known, but we think it results from the interaction of inheritance and environment. Inherited or genetic conditions often occur several times in a family, but most families have only one child with spina bifida. The role of inheritance in spina bifida is clearly shown only when large numbers of affected children are examined statistically. This role is more apparent when children with spina bifida and a closely associated birth defect, anencephaly, are statistically evaluated. Anencephaly is a very serious birth defect of the brain which is not familiar to most people because the children die at birth. Inheritance, however, does not entirely explain the occurrence of spina bifida.

Environmental factors are also thought to play a role, because spina bifida can be produced in animals by using various chemicals at critical times during the experiments. The animal mother's exposure to the substance must be at a certain time during the pregnancy, of a sufficient dose, and for an adequate length of time in order for spina bifida to occur. In animals these factors vary with each species (rats, guinea pigs, mice, etc.). Although this is true in animals, there is no evidence that any chemical or other agent causes spina bifida in man. However, it does seem possible that environmental factors may contribute to causing spina bifida in man. Perhaps a combination of genetic susceptibility and exposure to environmental factors leads to spina bifida in man.

Why Is Spina Bifida Considered Inherited?

In general, spina bifida and related disorders occur in approximately one among every 1,000 births. This is the so-called natural frequency of chance happening of the disorder. Therefore, one would anticipate that rarely brothers and sisters (siblings) of individuals having spina bifida would be affected by the same condition. On a random basis, if there were no genetic influence we would expect a spina bifida to occur in siblings at the general rate of one in every 1,000 births. However, this is not what happens. In general, siblings of children with spina bifida have a 4 to 5 percent chance of being born with a similar defect. This frequency (4 to 5 percent or one among every 20 to 25 births) is higher than the one among every 1,000 births that occurs in unrelated individuals. The increase is thought to be due to complex inheritance patterns that are not yet understood.

How Does Inheritance Work?

When the germ cells from two parents join to begin forming a baby, each brings with it genetic information. This information is carried by genes which guide the formation of the individual characteristics that the baby will have. Many characteristics are determined by only two genes, one from each parent. This is termed simple (monogenic) inheritance. However, some characteristics are determined by many genes. This is a more complex (polygenic) form of inheritance, and spina bifida appears to be inherited this way.

What Is Known About This Complex Inheritance?

Complex inheritance is not completely understood. The precise number of genes and how they interact to cause spina bifida is not known. Indeed, the whole concept of this type of inheritance is based mainly on the observation that some conditions such as spina bifida recur in certain families. Even though this pattern of inheritance is not thoroughly understood, extensive observations on large numbers of individuals permit an accurate statistical evaluation of risks in the families where spina bifida does occur.

Who Carries the Genes for Spina Bifida?

Individuals who have the genes for spina bifida are probably relatively common. These individuals are normal, and at the present time there is no way to detect that they carry the genes for spina bifida. They can only be identified when they have a child with spina bifida.

What About the Animal Experiments?

The experiments usually involve female animals who are pregnant. For instance, a female rat who has just been impregnated might be given a small amount of a chemical (aspirin for example) throughout the pregnancy. The baby rats would then be checked for spina bifida. This simple experiment could have many variations. The drug could be given to the mother rat before mating, at any time after mating, or only at certain times during the pregnancy. Other chemicals or different types of stresses on the mother rat could also be used. It is important to realize that in the experiments where the babies were born with spina bifida, the chemicals were used in much larger doses than those which humans normally take. Similar experiments could be done in other animals such as rabbits, hamsters, mice, guinea pigs, etc., to see if any of the changes found are special just for rats, or if they have broader implications which might relate to humans.

Although most experiments have been with female animals who are pregnant, the father or male animal may still have a significant contribution. When pregnant females are used for experiments, the effects are probably directly on the baby animals. However, when male animals are used, the experimental methods must affect the male sex cells so that the tendency for the infant animal to have spina bifida will be passed on during mating. It is much more difficult to show this relationship experimentally, and so far it is only speculation. However, fathers are more likely to be exposed to chemicals through their work; and although unproven, this may be important.

What Do We Know From the Experiments?

We have learned that the time during the pregnancy when the chemical or a stress is given is very important. A variety of experiments have shown that in order for certain chemicals to produce spina bifida they must be given at just the right time during pregnancy. If they are given too early or too late they will not cause spina bifida. This has led to the concept of sensitive periods during development of the baby. It is known that each organ system (brain, heart, kidney, etc.) has a special time during pregnancy when it is developing very rapidly. During this phase of rapid development an organ such as the brain is very sensitive to anything which might interfere with its growth. This may be one way that chemicals or other stresses act in leading to spina bifida. Unfortunately, the nervous tissue begins developing very early and continues to develop during the entire pregnancy. This makes it particularly susceptible. In contrast, an organ like the heart starts developing a little later and is completely developed by halfway through the pregnancy.

In animal experiments there are several methods of producing spina bifida. A colored dye called Trypan Blue produces spina bifida regularly in rats. Fortunately, humans are not commonly exposed to this dye. Vitamin A, which is in many of the foods we eat, can produce spina bifida when very large doses are given to animals at just the right time during pregnancy. Animals exposed to very large doses of x-rays, very low temperatures, or high concentrations of oxygen also can occasionally produce offspring with spina bifida. Some special viral infections in animals can cause spina bifida, as can very high doses of aspirin or insulin. Although these chemicals (Trypan Blue, insulin, aspirin, Vitamin A) and physical insults (x-rays, too much oxygen, low temperatures) can cause spina bifida in animals, all these agents must be used in doses or exposures far beyond what most humans ever receive. Indeed, the stress required experimentally is so extreme that it would probably seriously injure a human in other ways.

THERE IS NO EVIDENCE THAT ANY OF THESE AGENTS CAUSE SPINA BIFIDA IN MAN

Potato Blight

In 1971 a research investigator in England looked carefully at the geographical distribution of where spina bifida occurs most commonly and during which seasons of the year it is most frequent. He found that Ireland, where lots of potatoes are consumed, has a very high birth rate of children with spina bifida.

This reasearcher then proposed that perhaps something related to potatoes accounted for the presence of so many children with spina bifida. Potatoes periodically are damaged by a fungus called blight, and this was proposed as the possible cause. He also noted that more children with spina bifida are born after outbreaks of potato blight. This theory received a great deal of publicity in magazines and newspapers.

To prove the theory, an experiment was done in which pregnant monkeys were fed blighted potatoes. When some of their infants had nervous tissue defects like spina bifida, a large dietary study of human mothers was begun. In this study many pregnancies were carefully monitored while the mothers' diets were watched. Some mothers ate no potatoes. The result was that potatoes could *not* be shown to have any effect. Probably very few mothers ate blighted potatoes to begin with, and this theory has now been discarded.

What Occurs to Result in a Child With Spina Bifida?

The precise cause of spina bifida remains unknown, but complex (polygenic) inheritance is the most generally accepted cause of spina bifida. According to this concept, each parent of a child with spina bifida must carry a single set of genes for spina bifida. Both parents must contribute all of these special genes to that particular pregnancy. By pure chance most individuals with the genes for spina bifida will marry individuals who do not have spina bifida genes, and these couples will have almost no chance for a child with spina bifida. Again by chance, a small number of individuals with the genes for spina bifida will choose a mate who also has these genes. Such couples may have a child with spina bifida. Their risk of having a child with spina bifida will be approximately 4 to 5 percent, or one chance in every 20 to 25 pregnancies. This represents the change that both parents will contribute their complete set of spina bifida genes into the egg and sperm that combine to form the child. If a child with spina bifida is born, it is reasonable to conclude that both parents have the genes for spina bifida and the recurrence risk in subsequent pregnancies is again 4 to 5 percent. There is correspondingly about a 95 percent chance that one parent will contribute one or more of their normal genes and the child will not have the defect.

What Are the Chances It Will Happen Again?

For the common family situations, Table 3-I outlines what the chances are of having another child with spina bifida. Many other family situations are possible, but these are the most common ones. More distant relatives do not appear to have a significantly increased risk for having a child with spina bifida. However, if the parents are related, even distantly, the risk may be higher than usual.

Since so many situations are possible, each of which will modify predictions slightly, consultation with a physician for genetic advice is important. Parents who have a child with spina bifida should receive careful genetic advice, especially if they plan to have other children.

TABLE 3-I

Parent's Risk for Having a Child With Spina Bifida

Status Parents	Risk
Unrelated parents, no history in the family of spina bifida	1 in 1000 (.1%)
Unrelated parents who have one child with spina bifida	4 or 5 in 100 (4-5%)
Unrelated parents with two affected children	1 in 10 (10%)
One parent with spina bifida, no affected children	4 or 5 in 100 (4-5%)
One parent with spina bifida, one affected child	10 to 15 in 100 (10-15%)
One parent has a brother or sister with spina bifida	2 in 100 (2%)
One parent has nephew, niece, or cousin with spina bifida	1 in 1000 (.1%)

What Is Genetic Counseling?

Genetic counseling is a family health service which deals with the human problems associated with the occurrence of an inherited disorder in a family. The aim of counseling is to help the individual or couple understand: (A) the medical facts; (B) the risk of occurrence or recurrence of the disorder; (C) the choices which seem appropriate in view of their risk; and (D) how to make the best possible adjustment to the disorder.

Why Is Genetic Counseling Needed?

In general, birth defects are the primary reason for genetic counseling. They include all abnormalities present at birth and some inherited disorders which appear later in life. Some defects are caused solely by inherited factors, e.g. Down's Syndrome or Mongolism, some by environmental factors, e.g. Rubella or German Measles, and some probably by a combination of both, e.g. Spina Bifida. Our increased knowledge of genetics, improved techniques for diagnosis, and more effective therapy for many of these defects have prompted an increasing number of people to seek genetic services.

A couple's hopeful expectations may be cruelly disrupted by the birth of a child with a defect. This can create a crisis situation in the parents' lives. They may ask themselves: "What's wrong with me?" "What's wrong with us?" "What is the cause?" "Will it happen again?" Genetic counseling can reduce the anxieties and misunderstandings that individuals and couples may have about birth defects. It encourages the parents to ask questions and to air their concerns.

When Is Genetic Counseling Indicated?

Parents must first recognize that they need genetic counseling. This may come through personal concern within the family or may be suggested by a health professional working with them. Most genetic counseling involves the occurrence of a particular disorder in a child and the concern of the parents as to whether their future children might be similarly affected. Parents may also want to know about the risk for the affected child's offspring or the children of unaffected brothers and sisters. Couples who have no children as yet may be concerned about some aspect of their family histories. There are many possibilities, and counseling is indicated whenever prospective parents have concerns.

What Will the Counselor Need?

Before a family can be counseled, the nature of the defect in question must be precisely established. Often the diagnosis has already been made before referral and the couple wants information about the implications of the disorder for the family. The affected child and sometimes others in the family may need to be examined to confirm the diagnosis. The parents will usually be asked for the most complete and detailed family health history (family pedigree) that they can provide. This health history will go back two or more generations and may include the following:

(A) Age and health of each family member.
(B) Details of previous pregnancies in both parents and relatives.
(C) Details of any birth defects, serious illnesses, stillbirths or infant deaths.

What Does the Counselor Actually Provide?

The counselor's role is to provide the couple with (A) a realistic view of the situation including the nature of the birth defect already present in a family member; (B) the risk of the defect occurring again and what this means in practical terms; and (C) what options are available for dealing with the risk of recurrence. The counselor rarely recommends a particular course of action but rather helps the parents

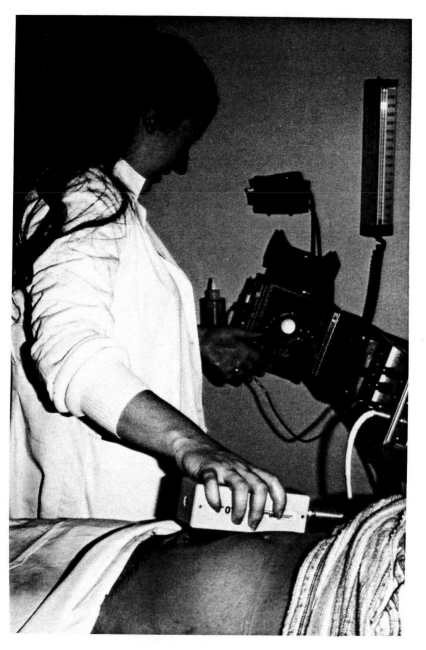

Ultrasound Examination.

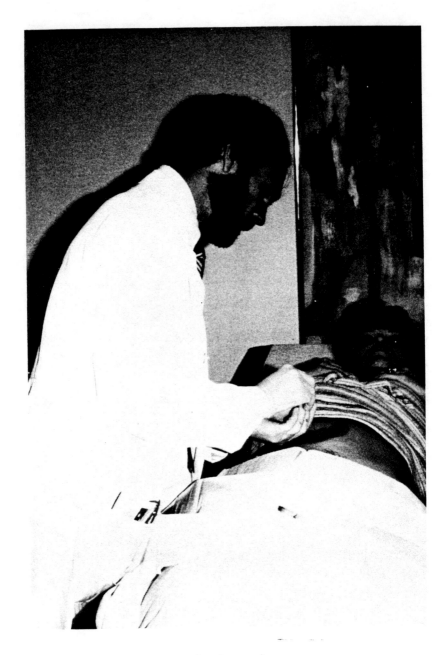

Amniocentesis.

make more informed choices if and when the need arises.

Can Spina Bifida Be Prevented?

Some families would like more children but feel unable or are unwilling to manage a second child with spina bifida. Can conception of a fetus with spina bifida be prevented? Complete prevention of spina bifida would require control of both inheritance factors and environmental factors, and this type of control does not exist. At the present time there is no known means of preventing spina bifida from occurring in the developing embryo and fetus.

However, the birth of a child with defects of the spinal cord or brain can be prevented. Nature takes the first step through what might be called a "biological filter." Nature frequently selects against developing embryos and fetuses which have such defects. The result is a spontaneous abortion or miscarriage which usually happens during the first three months of pregnancy. Almost half of these lost pregnancies have serious abnormalities of body development or abnormal chromosomes in their cells. The developing fetus who has spina bifida is subject to this filtering process, and some are spontaneously aborted. A second filter, prenatal detection, has been developed medically for detecting the abnormal fetuses that nature fails to reject.

What Is Prenatal Detection?

Prenatal detection refers to tests carried out during a pregnancy for the purpose of identifying certain abnormalities. It can detect some, but not all birth defects. In some cases, spina bifida can be detected. Detection is easiest for the fetus who is most severely affected.

When Is Prenatal Detection Done?

Prenatal detection cannot be done until the third month of pregnancy. However, by then the fetus has developed enough so that abnormalities can be recognized and there is enough fluid around the fetus so it is safe to obtain an amniotic fluid sample. It must be done before the fifth month of pregnancy so you can decide whether you wish to continue the pregnancy if it is an abnormal fetus. After the fifth month an abortion becomes increasingly risky for the mother.

Why Might Prenatal Detection for Neural Tube Defects Be Done?

As discussed earlier, parents are at an increased risk of having a child with spina bifida if: (1) one parent has spina bifida; (2) they have one or more children with spina bifida; or (3) they have close relatives with spina bifida. Each time you plan a pregnancy or are expecting a child, you should consider the value of prenatal detection and decide whether you wish to seek this service.

How Is Prenatal Detection Done?

Prenatal detection is performed by one of several procedures. One common procedure is called *amniocentesis* ("amnio" refers to the amniotic sac surrounding the fetus, and "centesis" means to perforate or puncture). The amniotic sac holds the fluid in which the fetus floats (amniotic fluid). This fluid can be sampled while the developing fetus is in the uterus. The fluid is obtained by passing a needle through the abdominal wall into this special sac and withdrawing a small amount of the amniotic fluid. This fluid looks like urine and is similar to blood serum in composition. The needle is placed by an obstetrician. It is painless and either local anesthetic or none at all is needed. It takes about one-half hour in the doctor's office, and you can go home immediately afterward.

How Is the Diagnosis of Spina Bifida Made?

Cells and chemicals in the amniotic fluid can be studied in the laboratory. Many substances are naturally present in the fluid, but the presence of other substances, or unusual amounts of some substances, may indicate an abnormal condition. Amniotic fluid normally contains a special protein called alpha-feto-protein. This protein is made by the liver of the fetus and is present in the fetal blood and spinal fluid. If there is a birth defect, such as a large spina bifida, the spinal fluid may leak into the amniotic fluid surrounding the fetus. This causes the level of alpha-feto-protein to rise above the normal level and indicates the fetus may have spina bifida. Other tests of cells and fluid are also sometimes helpful in diagnosing spina bifida or other conditions.

How Accurate Is This Test?

At this time, experience with this protein test shows occasional inaccuracies. These include both failing to identify a fetus with spina bifida and identifying a normal fetus as having a birth defect. About one out of five fetuses with spina bifida is not recognized by prenatal detection. Those missed usually have a spina bifida covered with skin, generally a less serious type, so there is little leakage of the protein into the fluid. The more severe forms of spina bifida are usually detected. A normal result from this test could reduce your risk of having a child with spina bifida from 5 percent to 1 percent or from one chance out of 20 to one chance out of 100. This remaining risk is mainly for having a child with a less serious type of spina bifida.

Different birth defects can occasionally cause the alpha-feto-protein to rise, but spina bifida is by far the most common cause. Rarely, a normal pregnancy will have an elevated protein level. This is usually explained by twins. Twins can be diagnosed by other tests which would be done if the protein level were high.

Other Tests That Also Help

Ultrasound is a test usually used along with amniocentesis. It provides a kind of picture of the fetus. Sound waves at frequencies above the range of human hearing are sent out by a scanner which is held against the mother's abdomen. Echoes from the various structures in the mother's abdomen (uterus and fetus) are displayed on a TV screen and photographed. No x-rays are involved. It is painless and harmless to both mother and infant. An outline of the uterus, the placenta, and the head and other parts of the fetal body can be seen. The outlines of two heads indicate twins. The picture may show abnormal development of the head. A high protein level in amniotic fluid along with an ultrasound picture showing a defect would greatly decrease the chances of any mistake. Movement of the legs can often be seen. When leg movement is present the more serious types of spina bifida are unlikely. Ultrasound technology is improving rapidly and better pictures of fetal structures should lead to more reliable detection of the many types of spina bifida in the future.

Other methods to test for spina bifida are being investigated. They may prove to be more accurate than those presently used.

It is possible that spina bifida in the fetus can be detected by testing a sample of the mother's blood. The special protein produced by the fetus also enters the mother's blood. Increased levels of this protein in the pregnant woman's blood, therefore, could identify the presence of an abnormal fetus. This test might serve as an easy and safe means for screening large numbers of pregnant women for fetal spina bifida. Such screening is presently being tested in some geographical areas, mainly in the United Kingdom.

Research on these techniques is progressing rapidly. All of the tests are designed to identify the fetus with a birth defect so that the family can decide if they wish the pregnancy to proceed.

Are There Any Risks to Prenatal Detection?

Many medical procedures carry some measure of risk for the patient. However, ultrasound is thought to be risk free as is the drawing of a blood sample from the arm. The risks of amniocentesis have been studied in a large number of women. The women were followed for the occurrence of complications to the mother, such as bleeding, infection, etc.; and those to the fetus, such as miscarriage, injury, and delayed development at one year of age. This study found equal numbers of these complications in both women who had amniocentesis and those who did not. Amniocentesis is thus generally considered to be a safe procedure which is appropriate to use when there is a significant risk of abnormality (about 1% or greater) to the fetus. However, the possibility of serious complications exists and amniocentesis should not be done without a good reason.

Is There a Risk With Abortion?

Abortion of an abnormal fetus involves some risk to the pregnant woman. It is difficult to make any general statement regarding how much risk, since the risk depends largely on the individual situation. Generally, the earlier in a pregnancy an abortion is done, the safer it is. You should, therefore, seek prenatal detection as soon as you know you are pregnant; even though amniocentesis cannot be performed safely until the third month of pregnancy. Should the tests indicate a birth defect and you choose abortion, there are several ways of inducing one. Each obstetrician will choose the method which they consider safest.

Is Prenatal Detection Useful If You Are Not Considering Abortion?

Prenatal detection is used to identify the abnormal fetus. This information might be valuable to you for reasons other than abortion. It could be done simply to give you information. Most often the results would be normal and very reassuring to you during the pregnancy. Occasionally, the test would show a fetus with spina bifida or some other defect. If you decided not to have an abortion, you would then have time to prepare yourself and your family for the birth of this child.

The Decision Is Yours

You might decide that prenatal detection is not of value or acceptable to you. The risk of having another child with spina bifida might not seem that significant to you, you might not want to know the outcome before the birth, or you might not approve of abortion.

You must decide if prenatal detection is meaningful for you. Your decision could include any of the alternatives suggested above. It is usually a difficult decision. The main issue is whether or not you would abort an abnormal fetus. Ninety to 95 percent of the time the results would be normal, and no further decision would be needed.

However, there is a 5 percent chance the results would not be normal. Some counselors in prenatal detection have thought that these tests should be done only if a couple has decided beforehand that they definitely would abort an abnormal fetus. Others think this requirement is unrealistic, since a prior decision might be changed in the face of the actual results. For this reason, a couple is now seldom required to state their decision before prenatal detection is done. But you would be encouraged to think through the issues and exchange thoughts with your spouse. You might wish to seek advice from other people such as friends, relatives, clergy, professional counselors, or your physician. These people could provide you with their opinions, and you could then consider them in forming your own.

If you decide to have prenatal detection, you and your obstetrician will need to evaluate your individual situation. Following this, it may be necessary to consult other specialists to obtain information on the availability, accuracy, and safety of the tests proposed.

There is one fact you should remember. Prenatal detection can help you to have children who do not have serious spinal cord and brain defects.

CHAPTER 4

BRINGING THE BABY HOME

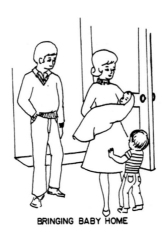

BRINGING BABY HOME

Figure 4-1.

How to Prepare

HAVING a child with spina bifida creates a new family situation. Some changes in your family life will be required. For some families, they are major modifications, and for others, minor. The extent and type of changes are unique to each family and depend upon many factors (family size, income, quality of communication between spouses, attitudes of those around you, etc.). At the base of these modifications is an adjustment of each family member's expectation of what the baby will be like. The family will have to come to recognize his special needs, as well as his good qualities.

Family preparation for the baby's homecoming should begin long before he leaves the hospital. You should consider the following factors which other parents of a newborn with spina bifida have found require attention.

Baby's Physical Care

One of your first concerns will be how to take care of your baby. If this is your first child, you will have questions about the kind of care

26

needed by all babies. A source of additional concern will be the extra tasks you may be asked to carry out because your baby has spina bifida.

There are many people who can help you in preparing for the homecoming. The nurses in the nursery can teach you about your baby's care. To insure that they do this, you may have to speak up and express your needs. There are certain times in the nursery which are better than others for teaching purposes. You and the nurses may need to plan a time in advance for these sessions.

If your area has a Spina Bifida Clinic or Birth Defects Center, there may be a nurse on the staff specializing in the care of these children. Upon request, she may be able to spend some time with you before the baby's homecoming.

Most areas in the country have a program of Public Health or Visiting Nursing. These are nurses based in the community who visit families at home. They can be of great support by visiting you and the baby periodically. Ideally you will meet the Public Health nurse before your baby goes home or at the time of discharge. This will give the nurse an opportunity to prepare for your child's and family's needs before making the first home visit. It is important to realize that even though this nurse may not have had contact with a great number of children with spina bifida, she can draw on her nursing background and consultations with the specialists to be of great help to you. You may need to request the services of such a nurse since a referral is not necessarily automatic.

Your pediatrician or other members of the specialty team caring for your child can be a wealth of information on how to care for your child. You will probably not feel entirely comfortable about providing this care until you actually give it a try. Asking questions and watching others demonstrate what you will need to do can give you a good head start.

The Other Children

Brothers and sisters of all ages need to know what is happening with their new baby brother or sister. Your explanations will depend upon the age of your other children.

With preschool children your emotional reaction to the baby's birth is more important than any explanation of spina bifida you might give. Since they are already particularly anxious about the new baby's arrival, they will be more so if you are unsettled. A preschool child is usually the baby of the family and being displaced from this favored spot presents some conflicts that you should recognize. It is perfectly natural for children of this age to openly express hostility toward a new baby. They may be direct and ask you to take the baby back to the hospital, or be indirect and demand attention when you are busy with the baby. One useful trick is to bring out their favorite book and read to them while you are feeding the new baby.

Regression or acting younger than their age is another common response to a new baby. For example, children who are toilet trained may regress to wetting their pants again. Most children eventually accept the baby, and in an effort to please Mommy and Daddy, they become very protective and concerned about the new baby. This is a normal response, but it can be accentuated when the new baby needs special attention.

Children from four to six years of age develop magical thinking. This is a wonderful feeling that you can do anything just by thinking it. Since most children have mixed feelings about new additions to the family, it is important to understand that, as a result of magical thinking, they may blame themselves for the baby's problems. It is important to reassure them that they could not and did not cause the defects.

With school-age children and adolescents you should give a simple explanation about spina bifida and encourage them to ask questions. Make it clear you are willing to discuss the baby's problems further. Do not overwhelm them with detailed information. Let them ask questions whenever they wish and answer them simply and honestly. They will set their own timetable for when they want to hear certain information.

Balancing Your Attention Among the Children

Rivalry among brothers and sisters and competition for the parents' attention is a normal developmental process for all children. The balance of attention parents achieve among their children is upset by the arrival of any new baby. However, the arrival of a disabled child may upset the balance even further, because the medical problems will require more of the parents' time and attention. Jealousy and resentment of the extra time required by the newcomer is typical. Wise parents will try to offset this expected occurrence by setting aside special time to spend with the other children. This does not necessarily have to be a lot of time, but it should be a time during which the other children can plan on having your undivided attention. You will find that time invested in this way will limit attention seeking behavior by the other children at those inconvenient times when you are trying to take care of the new baby.

An equal balancing of attention to all your children has other long-term implications. It is easy for parents of any child with a disability to become deeply involved in the child's care, become very protective and exclude other family members from this relationship. If this persists for very long, it is difficult to relieve the jealousies that result. This will tend to divide your family and further set your child with spina bifida apart from normal interaction with his brothers, sisters and possible friends. For the sake of all concerned, an early decision on how your parental time can be equally divided will be a wise preventative investment.

Relatives and Friends

By the time you are ready to take your child home and care for him, friends and relatives will expect you to know something about his condition. You will no longer be able to avoid their questions by responding, "I don't know yet." What should you tell them about the baby? A simple rule is to tell them the amount of information that you are comfortable answering. At first it may be difficult and upsetting to you to explain a great many details of the situation, and there is no need for you to do so. You may simply say the baby has a birth defect called spina bifida, where his spine has not developed correctly. This affects how he can use his legs, as well as other parts of his body. You may mention that he has required some surgery to repair the open spine and prevent other related problems. However, he is doing well and in many ways is just like any other baby.

Your relatives may be wondering if they too could be affected by spina bifida, or they may feel guilty in some way that their side of the family may be responsible for the birth defect. Relatives and inlaws can easily start blaming each other, causing additional stress for you. Neither side of the family is more responsible than the other. The professionals caring for your child can help answer a relative's questions about inheritance.

There are a small number of individuals who will have a great deal of curiosity about the baby's problem. They may ask a steady stream of annoying questions. Other people have a difficult time dealing with their own feelings or are clumsy in expressing them. Unfortunately they may pass their personal discomfort along to you. As you grow more relaxed and comfortable with your baby, you will find that you are either not bothered by the curiosity or insecurity of others, or that they become more relaxed with the situation because of your attitudes.

Changing the Daily Routine

The first change in the daily family routine may be when everyone is called upon to do their share. A joint effort will be required throughout the family to accommodate the needs of the new baby. Both parents will need to share responsibilities for the new baby with spina bifida and for the other children. The importance of dad sharing actively in caring for the child deserves emphasis, since it is a very large job for just one parent.

A special note of caution is needed for the natural tendency to depend heavily on your older children for help. Children of all ages need some freedom to grow up without being overly burdened with responsibilities. Certainly you can expect some help, but a balance of helping and free time is required. Often anger and resentment smolder in siblings who have been asked to sacrifice a great deal of their free time for the task of caring for the disabled child. Older daughters seem to be particularly affected by this problem.

Financial problems are another notable early concern. Comprehensive health care is expensive and you may worry that your current income, even with health insurance, will not be sufficient to cover the costs. You may consider working overtime or even taking a second job to supplement the family income. If you do, this will change how you interact in the family and may create added anxiety. If mother was working before the birth, she may not be able to return to the job as soon as anticipated. She may worry about all the extra things that need to be done for the baby and fear leaving him with anyone else.

With these aspects to consider, it is easy to understand how either parent can become confused with the new responsibilities. They might even feel guilty about shortchanging certain responsibilities or jobs. Simple rules to remember are:

(a) If both parents share the new responsibilities, it will be easier to maintain their own close relationship.
(b) Compromise is a key word when deciding what should be done and who should do it.
(c) Telling your spouse how you feel and openly discussing it will keep ties strong.
(d) As far as possible, all of the changes should blend in with family life the way it was before the new baby arrived. You will find that for the most part everyone will be happier if your new baby fits into the family, rather than the family completely changing to accommodate the infant.

Relief From Daily Pressures

In order to cope with life's extra challenges, you will actually have to plan time for relaxation. Take time to enjoy the company of your spouse, visit friends, attend an event, or just relax. You may find that scheduling relaxation, just like you would a dentist appointment, is the only way to insure that it will take place. Take time to share things as a couple and to continue intimate relations. Plan special weekends to get away so just the two of you can be alone. Often parents feel overwhelmed and shut out the new responsibilities and pressures. In this process they may exclude each other as a man or woman because of guilt feelings. Avoid becoming overly involved with responsibilities that could wait or that others might perform.

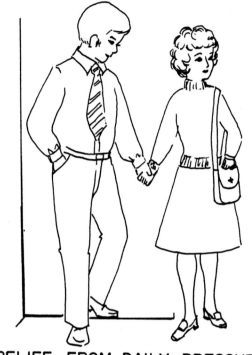

RELIEF FROM DAILY PRESSURES

Figure 4-2.

If you live near relatives and one of them feels comfortable caring for the baby, then take advantage of this support. You may feel more relaxed with that arrangement. You might search for a mature baby-sitter. Maturity is more important than age and even older adolescents from outside your family might be satisfactory. If you have a local Spina Bifida Association, they may have a listing of babysitters who feel comfortable caring for childern with special needs. If you are planning a long visit or a vacation, you might wish to investigate the respite care programs that many facilities operate. They can provide excellent care for a weekend or even periods up to several weeks.

Bringing your new baby home is a happy occasion even with all the special considerations. This is especially true if your baby has needed to stay in the hospital longer than usual. You should celebrate the homecoming according to any special family custom you might have. It will help bring the family closer together.

CHAPTER 5

FAMILY LIFE

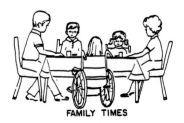

FAMILY TIMES

Figure 5-1.

The Parents

FOR many adults, rearing children is one of the most important and meaningful parts of life. Children are a source of joy, satisfaction, fulfillment, pride and love for their parents. They can be, at the same time, the source of responsibility, heartache, frustration and tension between their parents. This is true for all children, but having a child with spina bifida adds other dimensions to both the pleasures and problems of child rearing. Although many couples say that being the parent of a disabled child has strengthened their marriage, it is a rare couple who has not felt conflict and tension over the child with spina bifida. By first being aware that you can expect your child's special needs to be a source of extra stress you *can* learn to manage.

Sources of Stress

The possible sources of stress come from several directions. Some of the following are the common areas.

DIFFERENCES OF OPINION ON CHILD REARING. All parents have ideas on how a child should be reared. Usually they are based upon how their own parents dealt with them when they were growing up. Generally, it is difficult for both parents to be in complete agreement since they were reared in differing ways. There is room for greater differences of opinion in the case of a special child, since usually neither parent has been exposed to a disabled child growing up. Therefore, they have no model to copy and there may be more fear and worry about "doing the right thing." Genuine lack of knowledge and experience may turn questions like the following into sources of conflict:

What should we expect of our child?

Should we be strict or lenient?

What and how much should we do for this child?

RESPONSIBILITY FOR CHILD CARE. Mothers usually assume the largest share of a child's care, including taking the child to medical appointments. When you have a child with spina bifida, this responsibility is present around the clock and goes on for a longer time than for most children. Often mother has little energy left to enjoy the company of her husband, who may also be weary trying to keep the family financially supported and pay the medical bills. Today, more mothers are working as well, but they still retain a large share of the responsibility for child care.

HAVING OTHER CHILDREN. Differences of opinion on whether or not to have other children may occur. Parents may not understand their chances for having another baby with spina bifida, or differ in their opinions about taking the risk for another child (see genetics). In addition, if there is a feeling by either parent of an unequal burden in caring for the children in the family, it may affect their willingness to have a larger family. Disagreement on this issue can lead to increasing tension between parents, particularly in their sexual relationship.

AFFECTS ON SOCIAL LIFE. It is difficult to find babysitters willing and able to care for a disabled child. Therefore, parents may not be able to break away from these responsibilities, even for an hour or two of relaxation. In addition, neighbors and family may sometimes fail to include you, or even your family in an activity due to a mistaken notion about spina bifida. While your child is an infant, the extra responsibilities and fatigue may further curtail your social life. This can cause any parent to feel isolated and left out. There are also some recreational activities in which it is difficult to participate with a disabled child.

DIFFERENT TEMPERAMENTS. Fathers and mothers are individuals as well as a couple. They bring to their relationship different temperaments and have their own way of responding to stresses and life experiences. Having a child with spina bifida will affect each of them differently, and they will not respond in the same way to every aspect of a situation. For example, a father may try to conceal his feelings in order to be "strong for my wife." Yet his feelings may come out indirectly by his being irritated at the slightest provocation. A mother may talk about how badly she feels to relatives and friends, but avoid telling her husband because he "wouldn't understand." Both may feel hurt and become more distant from one another. Talking about how you really feel is a good start to keeping your relationship as strong as possible. A father might say "I should be strong, but I'm really concerned about . . . ," or a mother might say, "I hope you can understand how concerned I am about. . . . "

FINANCIAL PROBLEMS. The extra expense of caring for a child with spina bifida creates a financial strain for many families. In addition to medical care, there may be increased costs for transportation, alterations to your home, babysitting and other special needs. In order to meet these added expenses, the father may take a second job and the mother may go to work, or they may decide to do without things they otherwise would have been able to afford. Arguments then may focus on either picking an alternative or living with whatever decision is made.

How to Manage

Considering all these sources of stress, it is surprising to find that most families manage them satisfactorily and even superbly. The following are some of the techniques they have found to help them accomplish this.

PARTNERSHIP. There seems to be a crucial need to develop a sense of cooperation, of working together and sharing the care of all the children. This does not mean that both parents do all things equally, but rather that they both participate in the child's care by doing what each does best. For example, a father may wish to help his child with exercises while the mother takes care of toileting. Or, the parents may take turns in activities with the special child and then with the other children.

An especially important aspect of togetherness is in discussions with the medical personnel. While the mother may need to take the child for most appointments, both parents should make an effort to be present when new information is shared, important questions answered, or major decisions reached. If it is not possible for the father to be present at these times, he should be encouraged to call the physician to confirm information and ask his own questions. It places an extra strain on the parents' relationship if the mother is frequently in the position of relaying complicated, confusing, anxiety-producing information to the father. The same holds true when the father takes the child for medical care.

COMMUNICATION. An essential ingredient in any parental partnership is open, honest, understanding, respectful and loving communication. This is the way that differences can be aired, examined carefully, understood and resolved. Communication is hard work and may be painful at first. It is, however, one way that the pain can be eventually eased.

OUTSIDE HELP. All parents need both individual and shared interests apart from work and child care. Fathers and mothers can help one another by taking turns in caring for the children (so father can go bowling or mother play bingo). Many families have friends or relatives who are willing to learn about the care of a special child, so look

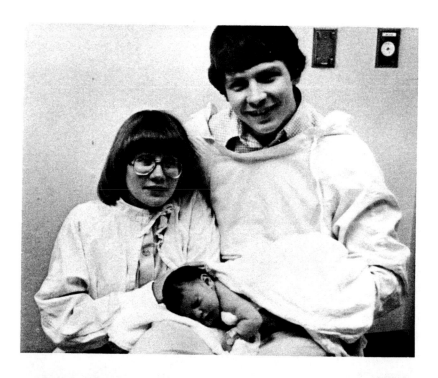

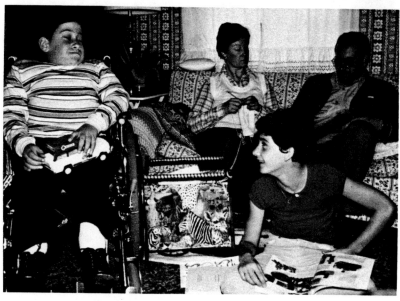

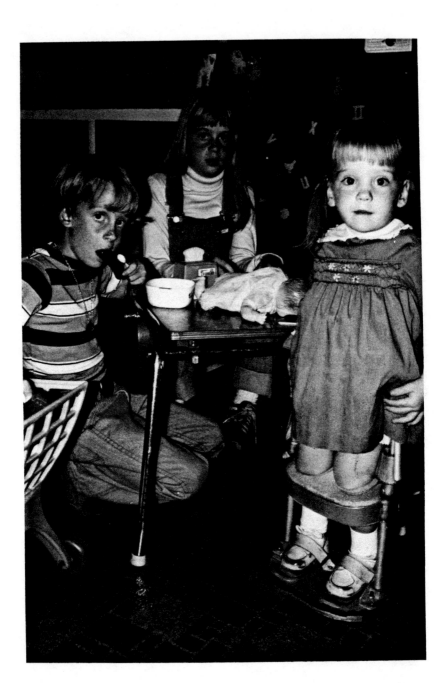

around you for willing people. A little time spent in educating a relative or friend about spina bifida could result in a source of life-long support.

Conflicts over how to manage your child may spring from lack of information or misunderstanding of the problems and needs. You need accurate information about spina bifida, your child's daily needs, and what you can reasonably expect. This includes information on the causes and risk of recurrence of spina bifida. Your Birth Defects Center, Spina Bifida Clinic, physician or other health care givers are excellent sources of this information. Some parents find it hard to remember what they want to ask when their child is being seen. Others feel hesitant to ask what seem like simple questions. Be assured everyone would much prefer that you ask. You may remember questions better if you write them down as they occur before your visit. Feel free to pull out your list and ask questions during the visit. If other questions arise or you feel confused after the visit, do not hesitate to call back.

Sometimes, even when you have the necessary information, you may still find there are differences of opinion over how to handle your child or over other family issues. At such times, counseling can be very helpful in working out a solution. Your family doctor or birth defects center may provide such counseling, or they will know of other places in the community where it is available. You may feel hesitant to admit there is a problem, either to yourself or anyone else. This is natural, but remember you are coping with a difficult situation. Timely assistance can help prevent prolonged tension, and that will be best for you, your special child, and other family members.

The local chapter of the Spina Bifida Association may be able to provide you with a wealth of emotional support (*see* parents groups). They may also have a used equipment pool, a collection of parent's practical suggestions for easing tasks of daily living, or a directory of competent babysitters.

The Brothers and Sisters

Parents' Concerns

Brothers and sisters are important members of all families. Parents are often concerned about how their other children will be affected by having a child with spina bifida in the family. Will the extra demands created by caring for a special child detract from their care of the other children? If this happens, the children could have adjustment problems. There is no reason to believe this must occur. Indeed, many families feel that their children who have a disabled brother or sister have benefitted emotionally and developed a greater respect for people with special needs.

How to Help Brothers and Sisters Adapt

The basic step is to develop a climate of acceptance for the new baby within the family. You can accomplish this in many ways. As soon as children feel free to talk, they will ask questions about their brother or sister, because differences are quickly noticed. Such questions should be answered simply, honestly and at a level your inquiring child can understand. The three-year-old who asks why his brother doesn't walk may only need to know that something went wrong before Johnny was born so he can't move his legs. The same questions asked by an eleven-year-old may require drawings of the spine and nerves and a deeper explanation. The same question asked by a sixteen-year-old may indicate a wish to know why birth defects occur and whether it will happen to his children.

When your child with spina bifida is hospitalized, the other children need to know why. They may be frightened about the hospitalization, even fear the death of their brother or sister. If you can encourage them to ask questions and express their ideas, you can lessen these fears.

Brothers and sisters will have many warm and loving feelings for the child with spina bifida, but they will also experience many negative emotions. All children·experience both love and hate toward their brothers and sisters, and the same is true when one has spina bifida. At times they may resent this special child's need for more parental attention. They may feel embarrassed by the attitudes and stares of others toward their disabled brother or sister. They may become angry at being asked to help with his care. They may feel lucky that they don't have such a problem. As a result they may feel *guilty* for having all of these thoughts. The impact of these feelings can be eased if you can listen patiently, reassure them you understand, and make it clear you still expect certain standards of behavior from them. "I know you wish I didn't have to do Sarah's exercises now, but I will read to you as soon as I finish."

Taking care of a special child requires extra time, and the other children may feel that they are being neglected. Their view will be partially correct, and it will be best if you can do something to decrease this feeling. One way is to plan special time with each of them individually. Select a time that is convenient for both you and the child and give him or her your undivided attention. You might play a game, take a walk, or just talk. The important part is that you express your interest in the child by making an effort to do some activity with them individually. In addition, you will want to plan some family activities like picnics in which everyone can participate.

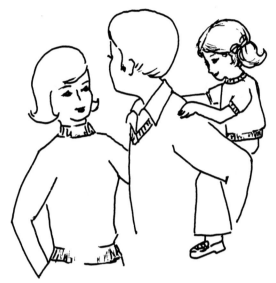

SPECIAL TIME FOR THE OTHER CHILDREN

Figure 5-2.

A source of conflict for some parents is how much to expect of the other children in the care of the child with spina bifida. All children should be expected to be helpful with one another and with household chores, but these responsibilities should not be beyond their capacities or encroach too heavily on their time for just being children. Brothers and sisters may help in some way by playing with their disabled sibling, doing some errands, learning to assist with dressing, or in countless other small ways. However, helping their disabled sibling should never be their major activity. Also, it should not become their main source of praise from parents. Every child needs to be valued as an individual and for himself, not simply for what he does to help out.

Another critical factor in helping brothers and sisters adjust to the child with spina bifida lies in your acceptance and response to the new situation. The children are looking to you as models for what to think and how to act. If you as parents attend to your marital relationship through partnership and communication and deal with the positive as well as negative feelings spina bifida triggers, you will be well on your way to promoting adjustment in your entire family.

CHAPTER 6

PROFESSIONAL HEALTH CARE

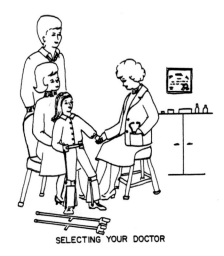

SELECTING YOUR DOCTOR

Figure 6-1.

PEDIATRICIANS and family doctors are concerned with growth and development, the prevention of illness, maintaining physical and emotional health, and the diagnosis and treatment of illnesses when they occur. All children need these types of services, but a child with spina bifida will find them useful more frequently. It is important that your child have a physician with a broad understanding of the child and the family. Although specialists may have a better understanding of various aspects of the child's problem, the family doctor should have the best overview.

Since children with spina bifida have special problems, your child's doctor will need additional knowledge about children with disabilities. Whether or not a doctor has the interest or ability to provide care to the child with spina bifida is dependent mostly on the individual. A frank discussion with him may help you understand if you can expect him to have the time or interest to work with you and your child.

The best relationship between you, your child, and your family doctor is based on mutual respect, trust, understanding, and interest. Since it may last over many years and will involve both planned and unplanned visits, you need to feel comfortable talking to him and asking questions.

Some doctors have limited contact with children who have serious birth defects and may be uncomfortable caring for children with spina bifida. It is very reasonable for you to ask your doctor how he feels about caring for your child. If he is uncomfortable, he may help you find a doctor who is more at ease in caring for children who have spina bifida.

Many physicians are not familiar with the most recent methods of caring for children who have spina bifida, but most are willing to learn. An early visit to the doctor without your child may help him to recognize the issues which are most important to you. He will also have an early start in seeking answers to your questions. Generally doctors are more able and willing to work with a child who has spina bifida if they have a team of medical and nonmedical health specialists who can help.

Whether your child's doctor is a pediatrician or a family practitioner should depend upon the individual physician and your confidence and trust in him. Both have training in the care of children. The training of the pediatrician is more intensive in child care, but the family emphasis may be equally important. In some offices, there may also be a pediatric nurse practitioner (PNP), a nurse who has special training in child care. Such nurses can be helpful in dealing with common problems and have access to physicians or other resources to help you handle some of the more difficult problems. Often it is easier to reach and talk to them than physicians.

What Can You Expect from Your Child's Doctor?

Your Child's doctor should:

Have a broad understanding of your family. The specialists may understand parts of your child better, but your doctor should have the best overview.

Listen to your concerns, discuss them with you, or refer you to the appropriate source to answer them. He may not know all the answers, but he should be willing to find them or help you find them.

Supervise the type of care which all children need (well-child care).

Provide advice or treatment for the usual types of childhood illnesses.

Be familiar with, or willing to learn, the signs and symptoms which suggest complications related to spina bifida.

What Can the Physician Expect from the Family?

The family should:

Provide him with information about the child. Be prepared to describe symptoms and relate what other doctors and personnel have said as well as the family's personal observations. When providing this information, be complete but brief. His background in medicine combined with the parents' intimate knowledge of the child is the best combination for assuring excellent care. He will need to see the child regularly in order to provide proper health care, and be familiar with his abilities when he is at his best.

Tell him of programs which might be available for your child or others. Programs in many communities change frequently and sometimes parents learn of the programs first.

Give him a chance to get the results of tests and communicate with others who can help when a problem arises. Remember that quality care takes a certain amount of time, and he has other patients. Being anxious may make it seem as if things are taking longer than they really are.

Understand that sometimes other patients may take priority. Such events may crop up at an inconvenient time for you, but should this become a continual problem, discuss it openly with him.

Openly discuss calling in a specialist if you feel especially concerned about some problem.

Let him know if you are pleased about the care your child is receiving. Physicians, like everyone else, need and appreciate kind words occasionally.

Aspects of Your Child's Care Which the Primary Physician Can Handle Best

Pediatricians and family practitioners are most skilled at providing well-child care. This includes the following common areas: childhood illnesses, feeding problems, weight control, emotional development, physical development, immunizations, and accident prevention. They may also be especially helpful in problems related to the spina bifida which are not being treated by specialists and in helping you understand what the specialists are recommending and doing.

Childhood Illnesses

You will find that when your child is small and cannot clearly communicate yet, you will be more likely to need your doctor's help to sort out common illnesses from more serious problems.

Call him for:

(1) *Fever over 102° F or a lower fever* (over 99° F oral or over 100° F rectal) which persists more than twenty-four hours. Most fevers in children result from viral infections, but the child with spina bifida runs a higher risk of kidney and central nervous system infections than other children. Thus, it merits closer communi-

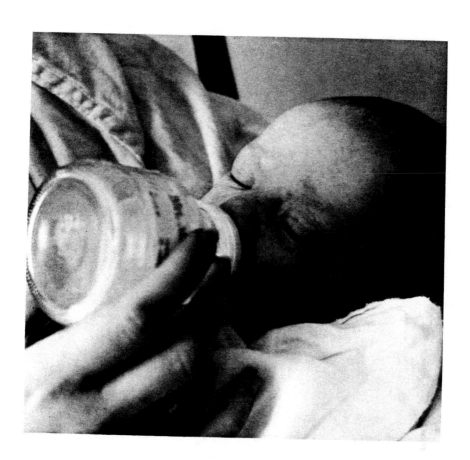

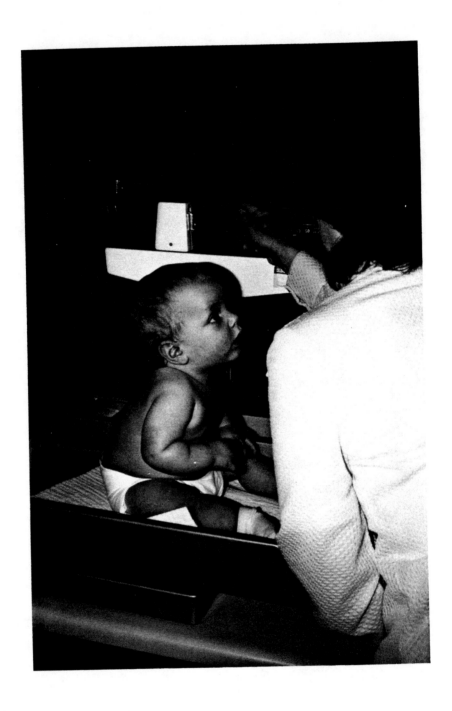

cation with your doctor when he is ill.
(2) *Lethargy and excessive sleeping.* These can be seen in any tired or sick child. However, if they are noticeably different from how your child acts with a mild illness or cold you need to check with your doctor. More serious infections or blockage of a shunt can also cause this.
(3) *Headache.* All children occasionally have headaches. If the headache is persistent or severe in a child who has a shunt, it could indicate a problem with shunt functioning.
(4) *Nausea and vomiting.* This is most often a viral stomach flu, but it can also occur with shunt blockage or urine infections.
(5) *Increased redness or tenderness* around a spina bifida skin defect which has not been repaired suggests infection and should be checked.

Common contagious illnesses are not likely to be more severe in your special child. Colds, sore throats, chicken pox, diarrhea and rashes may all occur and should be handled as in any other child. If symptoms are severe or associated with other signs of illnesses, your pediatrician should know.

Feeding Problems and Weight Control

All children need adequate nutrition to grow properly. Whether you nurse your baby or feed him formula is an early question that your doctors can help you answer. When to introduce solid foods and whether or not to add vitamins, fluoride, and iron are all questions which need to be decided on an individual basis.

Weight control is especially important in children with physical disabilities. Your doctor can help you evaluate your child's weight and assist you in keeping it at the appropriate level.

A child with spina bifida does have an increased need for foods that provide roughage in the diet in order to prevent constipation. Your doctor can help with advice on providing roughage in the diet and avoiding foods that may lead to constipation.

Emotional and Physical Development

All children need discipline. This is especially true for the disabled child who must depend upon others to help with his care. If expectations are not clear, then the child may not even carry out those tasks which he can perform. This can lead to serious problems of dependence. Your pediatrician can help you identify this or other areas which may lead to later behavior problems. He can also suggest methods of preventing or modifying these.

He can help you understand the ways in which your child's physical development is like other children. If the use of his legs is severely limited, he can also help you determine when you should encourage the use of extra devices — such as creepers, caster carts, etc. He can help you anticipate how to give your child a feeling of independence and self-sufficiency even if he needs extra physical help longer than other children.

Immunizations

All children need protection from tetanus, diptheria, whooping cough, polio, measles and rubella. Children with spina bifida are no exceptions. There are safe and effective vaccines that provide this protection. Sometimes vaccination against mumps is also indicated. Your doctor can guide you on when your child should receive these vaccines and also provide them.

Accidents

Your doctor can give you clues as to the different kinds of accident and poisoning risks your child may have at different developmental stages. In addition, one needs to be aware of other accidents that are more likely to affect your child with spina bifida. If your child has decreased sensation, he may not notice injuries to those parts of his body. Thus, he may develop frostbite in cold weather or pressure sores in shoes or braces without experiencing any pain. Even a fractured bone may go unnoticed unless swelling or a deformity is detected.

Your child should be encouraged to explore normally and be as active as possible. However, some planning to avoid accidents is also indicated. A bumper pad in the crib will prevent a leg becoming caught between the bars and causing a fracture. Older children can be taught how to examine their skin for early signs of pressure sores or frostbite. Safe, well-maintained equipment for ambulation will also help prevent accidents. These are just a few areas where a little planning may prevent later problems. You may discover other ways to prevent accidents by looking at your own child in his environment.

What to Do When an Emergency Arises?

Emergencies can arise and you should be prepared to take the appropriate steps if they occur. Some occasions are obviously life-threatening and require getting to a hospital quickly, usually by ambulance. Fortunately, such occasions are quite rare. More frequently, problems arise which are not so clear, and you may need help to determine if emergency care is really necessary. These situations are less urgent, and there is time to think about what should be done. Your child's physician can help you sort out these problems, and you should feel comfortable in calling him. Hospital emergency rooms do not function best in the role of sorting out the very sick from those who could be cared for less urgently. When they do this, there are very long waits.

You should try to be calm and sensible no matter what degree of emergency is occurring. A thoughtful, logical approach will be most beneficial to the child. Some events may seem like emergencies to families but may not be considered so urgent by others. It is best to contact your physician or a member of the health care team treating your child and discuss the situation with them. When you contact them, describe the problem carefully, but briefly, and state your concern and opinion. In the event you are unable to contact anyone, or if you are not satisfied with their opinion and continue to be very concerned about the child, then a trip to the hospital emergency room is certainly justified. When people are under stress, such as in emergency situations, it may seem that events are moving slowly or that others don't appreciate the urgency of the situation. This can then lead to the feeling that those individuals are not skillful or concerned enough to handle the situation. These are common reactions to stress and are usually untrue.

What Kinds of Emergencies May Happen?

The most common emergency problems in children with spina bifida are the following:

(1) Blocked shunt with hydrocephalus — There is usually lethargy, severe headache, vomiting or perhaps a stiff neck. This is a serious emergency, and if the child cannot be aroused, it is even more urgent to obtain neurosurgical help for him.
(2) Broken bones — These may occur in paralyzed legs and be apparent only by unusual movement, redness, or swelling.
(3) Serious urinary tract infection — There may be fever, back or abdominal pain, vomiting and nausea, or foul smelling urine.

SPECIALTY AND TEAM CARE

Each of your children deserves the best health care available. To see that your child with spina bifida receives it, you will need to understand the various ways that care can be provided. Then you can decide which health care system is best for your child and your family. There are two basic methods of health care — *general* and *specialty*.

General health care is that provided by pediatricians, family practitioners, and general medical doctors. All children need this type of care. Specialty health care, rather than viewing the whole child and his family, focuses upon a particular organ system (gastrointestinal, nervous, pulmonary, etc.) within the body. For example, a cardiologist is an expert on the heart and blood vessels, and a neurologist studies the nervous tissue and its disorders. Specialists are highly trained in a limited area, while generalists have a broader training with less depth of knowledge in each area. These terms, at times, become confusing, since a pediatrician is a specialist in treating children. However, physicians who practice general pediatrics actually provide a broad range of health care for the young. Both general and specialty health care will be needed by any child with spina bifida.

Since spina bifida affects many areas of the body (nerves, bones, bladder, etc.), you will need the help of several different specialists. Specialists in treating bones and joints (orthopedists), hydrocephalus (neurosurgeons), and urinary problems (urologists) are examples of specialties commonly needed by children with spina bifida. In addition, there are many other specialists who may be able to help your child at some point in time. One major decision you will need to make is how to coordinate the efforts of all the health care specialists whose care might benefit your child.

Coordinating your child's health care is a big task, but there are several ways this can be done. Since he will need a pediatrician (or other generalist) anyway, perhaps that individual could serve as coordinator. You and the doctor could then decide jointly when specialty consultation was necessary. This can be an excellent system. However, it requires that the physician be willing to assume this responsibility, that he will take the time and make the effort to coordinate the care, and that he will and can communicate ideas and opinions between all those involved. This is a sizeable task, and some physicians are not prepared to assume it. If you choose this system, you should discuss it openly with your doctor and be certain he is agreeable.

Another method is for you, as the parent, to arrange visits with the pediatrician and the individual specialists. In this way, you will serve as coordinator and be responsible for relaying some information between the various parties. You will be required at times to decide when treatment or a particular specialist is needed. This places a big responsibility upon you as parents and is not recommended. Occasionally families find this system adequate, or the only method available to them.

Team Health Care

A third type of arrangement is to utilize a health care team. Since most team care is located in large medical centers, a team may not be readily available to everyone. When a team is available, it has several advantages. The specialists who participate as team members will have a special interest in spina bifida, be knowledgeable about it, and have experience in its treatment. Because these specialists routinely see large numbers of children with spina bifida, and have access to the latest advancements in treatment, a team can provide both expertise and experienced care. A team can also improve the coordination of your child's care. Often the opinion of one specialist directly affects the ideas or recommendations of another, and it is helpful when they work closely and can communicate directly. A coordinated effort by all the specialists is required if your child's special needs are to be met. Another benefit of the team approach is that they usually include members who specialize in helping with social, emotional, and daily management issues. Medical specialists sometimes do not address these issues, but they can be a major source of strain within the family. These team members, working together, try to address as many issues as possible during a visit, and then communicate their thoughts to your child's primary physician to provide a total health care program.

Health care personnel who work as team members feel the benefits this care brings to the children and their families is important. They feel the opportunity to discuss difficult management problems with colleagues whose expertise is in other areas improves the child's overall health care, and that this interchange improves everyone's understanding of the family's total needs. A team setting is also an opportunity to learn and to teach. Teaching helps to develop proper attitudes toward the disabled among students and physicians in training.

As in any system, there are some concerns which team care raises. Initially, it may appear that team care is more expensive. Bills for team care are larger than for a single doctor's visit, because the cost usually does not reflect only the physician's fees. The cost of maintaining other team members who may be working on your child's behalf at many other times may also be included. Teams are generally expensive to operate, but only a portion of the true cost is usually billed to families. Private foundations or federal grants often subsidize the remainder. Team evaluations do require more time than evaluations by a single person. This is because many team members may see a child, time is usually spent in communication between staff members, and, since most teams are in large medical centers, there may be students present. A team visit may involve an entire afternoon, but it may also eliminate several trips to various offices at different times. You may save both time and money by making a single visit to one location.

Defining Who Needs to See Your Child

You could personally decide when you would like the services of any specialist, but many parents find that decision places a large responsibility on them and is difficult to make. Working with a team relieves some of this strain. An effective health team should understand your needs and those of your child and family well enough to effectively direct you to the care your child needs. Some parents are grateful for this, but others feel a loss of control or even freedom of choice. Whatever health care program you select, find the program that works best for you and your child.

Working with Your Health Care Provider

The basis of any good relationship rests in the quality of communication between the participants. Feeling comfortable in the presence of individuals who care for your child helps the flow of communication. You should select people whom you respect and with whom you feel comfortable speaking. This may give you a good start, and these people can help you contact others who may be helpful. Although you may feel more comfortable with a health care provider as time passes, you may have to make an active effort to accomplish this.

In working with any health care provider, you must be willing to share your ideas as they arise. Unless you share your personal concerns and opinions with others, they may remain unknown. Sharing your concerns can lead to a better understanding of what you can realistically expect treatment to accomplish. This in turn can prevent misunderstandings which might delay or interfere with your child's care.

When problems or crises arise and stress mounts, some individuals respond with anger. These feelings may be directed at or simply spill over onto the health care providers. There may be aspects of the child's care which have not gone as anticipated. Mistakes may have occurred or your child may have become ill at a particularly stressful time. No matter what causes the anger, you should try to express your concern so that others will be receptive to hearing your viewpoint. If you feel upset, either about the care or with a particular professional, an open discussion may be helpful. Try to be tactful and constructive. If you are critical of treatment or an individual, try to also suggest ways to improve the situation. If this brings no resolution, you can then consider another source of health care; but do so only after careful consideration and efforts to work out your grievances. Any change which disrupts the continuity of your child's health care risks overlooking important aspects, and generates frustration for all concerned. Shopping around among health care givers is rarely beneficial to your child. Spina bifida is a complex problem, and times will almost certainly arise when either you, the health care givers, or both, will feel stressful and frustrated.

In order to understand your interactions with other individuals, it is helpful to recognize your own feelings. This includes your feelings about relationships at home and work, as well as with your health care providers. If you have difficulty doing this, then professional guidance, such as from a social worker, may be helpful. Many parents of children who are disabled find counseling beneficial, and you should not be embarrassed or ashamed to ask for someone to speak with you. You should also be receptive to observations about your child's success in handling problems. Social and emotional issues are sometimes particularly sensitive areas, but a request for help can represent a real strength on your part. Providing your child with the best possible environment in which to grow is everyone's goal, and early attention to any problem area may prevent more serious difficulties later.

When you do contact your child's health care givers, consider how you can most profitably use their time. Prepare your questions in advance or even make a list of your questions or concerns. This will save time and assure that all your questions are answered. Whoever coordinates your child's treatment can then either provide answers or help you decide who might best answer a specific issue. Working together, you can provide your child with the best health care.

THE ROLE OF THE DENTIST

The teeth of children with spina bifida are no different than the teeth of other children. The care should, therefore, be the same. In children who are disabled, general care of the teeth may be overlooked until dental problems arise. This is unfortunate, because teeth play an important role in health, and dental disease can be prevented.

Teeth are the first step in the digestive process. They are important in clear speech and improve your personal appearance and smile. If we look good, we feel good! A feeling of well-being is an important part of good health, and good health helps us perform to the maximum of our ability.

When Do You Start Dental Care?

The first teeth usually appear at about six months of age. Dental care should begin at this time. This consists of brushing the teeth and gums with a soft toothbrush and water one or two times a day. It is important that dental care become a daily routine.

The child's first visit to the dentist should be at the age of two years but no later than three years. Prior to, and between dental visits, one should regularly look at the child's teeth. If there are any problems, such as cavities, the child should be taken to the dentist as soon as possible. The normal time between regular check-ups should be about six months.

Selecting Your Child's Dentist

The same care should be taken in selecting a dentist as when you chose your child's physician. You should try to find a dentist who is interested and willing to treat your child and will provide both psychological and dental care. Pedodontists are dentists who specialize in dental care for children, and they have special training in dental care for the disabled. Some general dental practitioners also care for children including children with disabilities. Before making any dental appointment for your child, discuss your child's disability with the dentist.

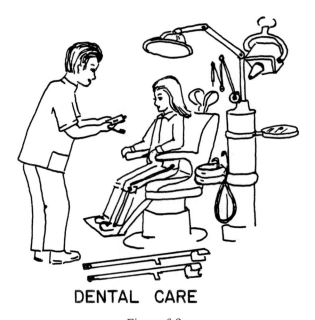

DENTAL CARE

Figure 6-2.

Prevention of Dental Disease

A healthy tooth is always preferable to one that has been repaired. Practicing prevention in the home requires a commitment of time and effort on the part of the parents.

Tooth decay (or dental caries) is a disease that occurs when three basic factors come together. The first factor is a susceptible tooth, the second is bacteria, and the third is sugar. All teeth are susceptible to decay, but those with pits or fissures in the biting surface are especially likely to decay. Bacteria are normally present in the mouth, but good oral hygiene controls the amount of bacteria on the teeth. Sugar in the diet helps the bacteria to live and grow. From sugar, bacteria makes a sticky material called plaque. Plaque protects the bacteria and enables them to stick to the teeth. The bacteria also makes an acid which can dissolve the enamel on the teeth and, thus, allow bacteria to enter the teeth and cause decay.

Babies who have a bottle at nap time or bedtime are at very high risk for tooth decay. If the child falls asleep with a bottle of milk or juice in his mouth, the liquid may remain on the teeth during the entire nap or throughout the night. This can cause such serious damage to the teeth that they often cannot be repaired and must be taken out. It is a tragic situation which can be avoided by not giving a bottle at bedtime. If the bottle must be continued, fill it with tap water or substitute a pacifier.

If we break the combination of these three factors — susceptible teeth, bacteria and sugar — we can eliminate decay.

Cleaning the Teeth

Removal of the bacterial plaque can be accomplished mechnically with a toothbrush and dental floss. When your child is old enough to want to brush his own teeth, this should be encouraged. Use of toothpaste may make brushing more pleasant. Young children need to have their teeth brushed by a parent, and older ones should have their brushing checked. Most children learn to accept toothbrushing once it becomes a part of their daily routine.

It may be difficult to see the plaque, but disclosing solutions color the plaque (usually red) and make it visible. They can be bought in most drug stores. In small children they can be painted over the tooth surfaces with a cotton swab, and older children can swish a few drops around in the mouth, or chew and swish a disclosing tablet.

Once the plaque is colored, the brushing can begin. Toothpaste is *not* recommended. Simply wet the toothbrush with water. Once the teeth are clean and no more red-stained plaque can be seen, they should be flossed. This is necessary because the toothbrush cannot clean between the teeth. Unwaxed floss is recommended, and a floss holder may make the task easier. The floss must be gently slipped between the teeth and the surfaces polished.

Complete plaque removal should be done once a day, and the teeth should be brushed after every meal. When older children brush their own teeth, one of the brushings should be supervised. The best time for supervised brushing is at night, just before bedtime, as a part of the child's nightly bedtime ritual. Between brushing and bedtime your child should not eat or drink anything except water.

Controlling Sugar in the Diet

Eliminating as much sugar from the diet as possible is another way to prevent decay. You should avoid foods high in sugar content, especially between meals. Substitute fresh fruits and vegetables, cheese, nuts, popcorn, corn chips and the like. Sugarless soft drinks and chewing gum are also helpful. Give your child foods that require chewing and eliminate soft and sticky foods. Sweets which are part of a meal are less harmful than those given as between-meal snacks, especially if the teeth are brushed after meals. Your dentist can give you other suggestions on how to reduce the sugar in your diet.

Fluorides

Fluoride is now considered essential for teeth. Fluoride in the water supply is the most effective way of reducing tooth decay; and if your water supply is fluoridated, your child is probably receiving adequate fluoride. If your water does not contain enough fluoride, your dentist can prescribe supplemental fluoride in the form of tablets, drops, or rinses. In addition, topical fluoride applications by your dentist can further strengthen the teeth and make them less likely to decay. If your child uses toothpaste it should contain fluoride.

Fluoride is very effective on the smooth surfaces of teeth, but it is less effective on the biting surfaces. Pits and fissures on these surfaces act as small traps for bacteria and food, and they are too small to be cleaned by a toothbrush. In order to reduce decay on these surfaces, a fissure sealant must be used.

Fissure sealants are plastic materials which are painted over the biting surface of a tooth. They harden into a plastic "shield" which seals out food and bacteria. They are easily applied by your dentist without discomfort or anesthesia, and they greatly reduce the chances of decay formation. Sometimes they may need to be reapplied when the child is older.

The Goals of a Preventive Dentistry Program

Good oral health means better health in general for your child. A good program to maintain oral health is designed to reduce tooth decay and gum disease. It will require some daily effort, but most aspects of the program are easily worked into a family's routine.

Dental Treatment for Children with Shunts

Although a physical disability may modify the performance of dental treatment to a child with spina bifida, the actual treatment is the same as for other children. However, special precautions must be used for children who have shunts which enter the bloodstream (ventriculoatrial shunts). This is necessary since some dental treatment, including some preventive care, may cause bacteria to enter the bloodstream. The body normally protects us from these bacteria; but if there is a shunt draining into the bloodstream, it is possible for this to become infected. This is unlikely to occur if the shunt does not enter the bloodstream, such as the ventriculoperitoneal (VP) shunt.

The precautions needed are antibiotics. These are given to the child with a shunt before the dental treatment and continued for about two days afterward. This protects the child from any bacteria which may enter the bloodstream. Commonly, one of the penicillins (dicloxacillin) is used if the child is not allergic to it. If there is an allergy to penicillin, then another antibiotic may be substituted. The penicillin is started about one hour before treatment, and the dosage used for protection is similar to that recommended with penicillin by the American Heart Association for children with heart problems. Your dentist should be familiar with the dosage.

If you have any questions about your child's dental health, discuss them with his dentist. He will appreciate your interest and the opportunity to help.

CHAPTER 7

COMMUNITY RESOURCES

IN most cities there are a variety of community services which may be useful to a family who has a child with a disability. Some of these services will be specifically for disabled children. However, other services may be more general and make no distinction in eligibility. What is important is that help and support are usually available. Chances are that someone before you has also needed the same things you do.

What Types of Services Might Be Useful?

The needs of each child or family will differ depending upon many factors. Among these are the child's specific disability, age and intelligence, and the family's unity, resources and experiences. However, some common services that may be useful are help with medical or home care, special educational or recreational opportunities, counseling and child care or babysitting.

Where to Start

Each community is different, and it may take some time for you to identify the available resources. Be persistent and do not get discouraged. Speaking with your child's health care providers, or parents of other children with disabilities, are two good places to begin. Explain to them what you are seeking and establish if they are familiar with programs which provide these services. The telephone book is another good place to begin. Some communities have an information or referral service, often called a "hotline." The people who run this may be able to help or may suggest other places to check. If there is a local Birth Defects Center or Spina Bifida Clinic, the various team members can probably be helpful. Other communities may have progressed to a drop-in center, perhaps sponsored by the United Way or Community Chest. There may be a parents' group for families whose children have spina bifida; but parents' groups for children with other disabilities can also be useful. Radio talk shows are remarkable sources of information, especially when the audience can call in and provide tips. Parent groups of all kinds can be contacted. Do not overlook other health-related community groups like the local branch of the Cerebral Palsy Association or even the Cancer Society.

52

Listed below are a few categories and suggestions as to where you might start looking for help.

1. *Help With Health Care*:
   Your family doctor and office nurse or nurse practitioner.
   Visiting or Public Health Nurses.
   The Public Health Department (city, county, state).
   Professional groups (Medical Society, Nursing Association, or Physical and Occupational Therapy Associations).
   Home Care or Homemaker Programs.
   The Red Cross.
   The local hospital or medical center.
2. *Daytime Programs and/or Recreation*:
   Day Care Centers.
   Nursery School Programs (public or private).
   Project Head Start.
   YWCA or YMCA.
   Special Programs sponsored by United Cerebral Palsy, Association for Retarded Children, Easter Seal Society, Rotary, Kiwanis, Lions, or various women's groups.
   Local church or temple programs.
3. *Counseling*:
   The local Family Service Association. (These are often run by religious groups such as the Catholic Family Service or Jewish Family Service.)
   Mental Health Centers.
   Hospital or County Social Service offices.
   Parent groups which sponsor professional group sessions from time to time.
4. *Educational Testing for Your Child*:
   Public School Guidance departments.
   Private testing services. (First be sure they are approved by professionals in the area.)
   Mental Health Programs.
5. *Financial Help*:
   The County Health Department, Department of Social Services, Medicaid or welfare offices.
   Your insurance company can help you understand the coverage provided in your policy.
   Your bank has financial advisors who can help with situations such as unanticipated medical bills.
   The hospital billing office to discuss a plan of payment that fits your means.

Local Parents' Groups Deserve Special Consideration

There comes a time when most parents feel, "No one really understands what I am going through. Everyone has been helpful, but they aren't the parents of a child with spina bifida." The opportunity to share problems with someone who has already faced the challenge, or who is facing it at the same time as you, is often helpful. Some parents would like to talk with other parents soon after they bring their baby home, while others prefer to wait awhile. How ready you are for this type of experience and information is something only you can decide.

What Types of Contact Are Available?

To start you may wish to meet another parent who has a child with spina bifida. This type of personal contact can be very supportive and reassuring. Meeting another family requires consideration of their needs as well as your own. Such a meeting may be arranged by the health care team, your child's physician, or by a local group. Spina Bifida Parents' Associations are being formed across the country. They are modeled after groups for parents of children with other disabilities. *The Spina Bifida Association of America* (SBAA) was formed in 1972. The purpose of the organization is to assist parents to achieve the maximum potential for their children. The SBAA holds annual meetings where parent representatives come together to learn about new methods of treatment, to work for better care in local communities, to improve legislation for the disabled, and to have an opportunity to share ideas. If there is not a local Spina Bifida Association in your area you may find support from similar organizations for parents whose children have other disabilities, or you could consider forming a group.

What Do Parent Groups Do?

Parent groups provide support and help for families through understanding, companionship and advice. Since spina bifida affects children of families from every walk of life, most organizations have a diverse membership and develop a mixture of programs. Some groups can help you find and use the services your child may need.

The various types of activities sponsored within parent groups are a testimony to the desire they have for providing support to one another. Too often, the arrival of a child with spina bifida causes a family to isolate itself and disrupts previous social activities. Involvement with a parents' group can encourage socialization. The following list outlines some of the activities a parents' group can engage in:

1. *Hold Regular Meetings.* These can be used for educational talks to share knowledge of local services or present information of interest to the members such as recent methods of care. Meetings

are also a good time to renew friendships or establish new ones.

2. *Sponsor Family Programs.* Family dinners, special parties for children, organized swim programs or other recreation activities can be enjoyable and supportive to members. These can help families with younger children to understand the importance of including all the family in activities and maintaining a normal, although modified, life-style.

3. *Provide Role Models.* Adults who have spina bifida and are leading independent lives can furnish valuable leadership and serve as role models for the younger children. Parents of older children with spina bifida can also be models for those with younger children.

4. *Improve Health Care.* By working with local health professionals, they can assure that the children receive the best care possible.

5. *A News Letter.* A regular news sheet can help parents learn of new developments and reach out to those unable to attend all the meetings.

6. *An Equipment Pool.* This can help families save money by passing equipment or certain homemade objects on to other children.

7. *Community Projects.* An organization can effectively become involved in many community activities. It can help to improve local services. It can also make citizens more aware of the abilities the disabled possess.

Is a Parents' Group for You?

Many parents have found comfort and support by joining a parents' group. Some parents, however, are simply not comfortable with the group approach, and this individuality should be respected. Persistent attempts to draw them into the group may produce anxiety rather than support. Other families will find that time or distance makes it difficult for them to participate.

The needs of individual parents or families usually vary with their own interests, personalities, life situations, and child's disability. If the interest and emphasis of the group corresponds to that of the parents, then a great deal of benefit can be derived from participating. Whether you should participate is a personal decision only you can make.

The Professional's Role in a Parents' Group

Parents' groups provide an aspect to the child's care that professional resources cannot. Parents, after all, have personal experience with spina bifida. Similarly, the professionals have knowledge and skills that parents lack. It seems wisest that professionals have some role, either as advisors or active members. Working together will help both groups be more effective in providing for the welfare of children with disabilities.

CHAPTER 8

FINANCIAL HELP

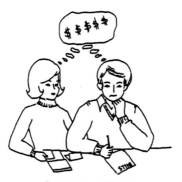

FINANCIAL CONCERNS

Figure 8-1.

WHILE your immediate concerns will be for your child's welfare, you must prepare for the extra cost of his health and related care. Those families with very comprehensive health insurance may not have too much of a problem managing health care costs. Others with average or less coverage may be faced with accumulating bills which their insurance does not cover. Fortunately, most families carry insurance for care which requires hospitalization. The majority of insurance policies cover the bulk of the cost for procedures and professional fees accumulated during an inpatient hospital stay. Problems arise when help is needed to pay for care received on an outpatient basis. Coverage for visits to your physician's office, Spina Bifida Clinic, or outpatient x-rays and other special procedures may not be included under your policy. Since your child will receive most of his medical care as an outpatient, significant expenses may accumulate in this way. You should contact your insurance company or the benefits office where you work to check on exactly what coverage your policy provides.

Hidden expense items are another source of financial drain. These items can be costly, and most are not covered by insurance, no matter how thorough your policy. Examples of hidden expense items are: transportation for frequent trips for health care, special clothing, braces, diapers, food supplements and architectural modifications to your house when your child grows older.

57

What Are Sources of Financial Help?

In nearly every state, there is some type of program which offers financial assistance to families of children with disabling conditions. The programs have different names and usually require that your financial status and income be screened. Who qualifies financially for assistance varies from state to state. The following are some possibilities for financial assistance which you might investigate, depending on your particular circumstances.

MEDICAID. Medicaid will pay for health care for families with very low incomes or none at all. This federal- and state-funded program usually covers both inpatient and outpatient fees. To determine your eligibility for this program you must apply at your local Department of Social Services or Health.

AID TO PHYSICALLY HANDICAPPED CHILDREN. This particular program is highly variable depending on where you are residing. The federal government mandates that states set aside some money to assist in providing the care that is required by disabled children. The amount of money available through this program varies from state to state and county to county. Each local area decides the items and types of programs they can underwrite, thereby leading to further variations.

An example of what is available through one program would be the one in Monroe County, New York. Expenses picked up by this program are shared 50 percent by the county and 50 percent by the state. The county portion is managed by the health departments located in each major city of the county. The state portion and overall directorship comes from the:

Bureau of Medical Rehabilitation
Empire State Plaza
Towers Building
Albany, New York 12237

The Monroe County program attempts to pay for diagnostic evaluations and items such as special equipment, medications and certain outstanding hospital bills. It also supports some of the health care fees for children receiving care in the local Birth Defects Center.

Eligibility for this program is determined when parents apply at the various local offices. Generally, parents can have a greater income than is acceptable for some other programs and still receive assistance on this program. A specific request must be submitted for each item for which help is desired. This program also funds some centrally located clinics and underwrites fees for children seen by certain specialists. Your local public health office, state or county health department, public health nurse or school physician should be able to provide you with information on how this money is utilized locally.

Another use for this fund comes from the federally mandated program (Public Law 94-142), which says that each state must make an effort to seek out and diagnose children with disabling conditions. This program does not provide for on-going care after the children are found. How each state "finds" its disabled children varies also.

This service should be available regardless of a family's income. The number of cost-free visits to a specialist or center to ascertain the nature of the problem also varies from state to state. In Monroe County, three initial visits to the local center are funded for particular children in search of a diagnosis.

SUPPLEMENTAL SECURITY INCOME (SSI). This is a federal program which makes monthly cash payments to disabled adults or to families of children who do not have much income or other assets. A parent or guardian can apply for a child at the Social Security office and obtain a decision on whether their child is eligible for this type of help. This financial help may be available for those residing in institutions under certain circumstances. Those preparing to leave an institution may be eligible for SSI as a source of income. A child cannot receive payments and still take part in the program of Aid to Families with Dependent Children (AFDC-welfare). But if a child is eligible under both programs, parents can choose whichever one best suits the family. In many states, a person eligible for SSI is also eligible for Medicaid. Further information on this program is available through your local Social Security office.

SLIDING SCALES. Many health care programs have a sliding fee schedule. This means that you are billed according to your income and ability to pay. Do not be bashful about inquiring.

PHILANTHROPIC GROUPS. There are many charitable organizations around the country. Some deal in sizeable sums and others are small operations. Each decides how they want to spend their money. Some may prefer to fund research into the cause of birth defects, but others are interested in helping families pay for expenses already accumulated by a disabled child. Parents simply have to be alert to local resources such as these.

How to Work Through the Red Tape

Patience, persistence and the willingness to ask questions are the three most important qualities in tracking down financial help. Be courteous but firm when dealing with people in the various government or billing offices. If you feel you are getting the "run-around" or the person seems to be poorly informed, speak to the supervisor or whoever is at the next higher level.

Whenever speaking to anyone about programs, ask if there is any written material available. Be sure you write down the names of the people with whom you talk. You may need to return someday or refer others to this person.

Be careful to keep a list of all expenses associated with your child's health care. Most are tax deductible even if they are not covered by your insurance policies. Try not to allow your bills to pile up before asking for help.

If you have difficulty finding help or knowing what to do, you should look for some emotional support and practical tips. These may be obtained through other parents who have experienced similar problems or the staff where your child receives his health care. Above all, remember that financial stress is a major source of family problems. By planning ahead, setting realistic priorities and getting sound advice, you should be able to avoid a multitude of unpaid bills. Not only will you feel more free to seek the health care your child needs, but you will spare yourself and the whole family unnecessary emotional stress.

CHAPTER 9

SOCIETY'S RESPONSE
TO THE DISABLED

What Will Others Think of Your Child?

THE attitude of society toward people who are disabled is becoming increasingly positive. For many years, society treated disabled individuals as people to be feared. This attitude may have arisen from the misconception that whatever caused the problem might be catching. Leprosy was one of the earliest identified disabling conditions, and perhaps this fear began because lepers were thought to be contagious. The natural conclusion that people drew was probably that all disabling conditions could be transferred to others through close contact. Avoidance of the disabled seems to have originated very early.

Today our understanding of birth defects and disabilities is more scientific. Nevertheless, misunderstanding is still prevalent in our modern-day society. We still avoid what we do not understand. In addition, our imagination about the nature of the problem is usually more exaggerated than warranted by the facts.

Until recently, an institution or other special setting was thought to be the best way to deliver services to the disabled. Unfortunately, this segregation prevented society from working, playing and learning about the disabled. Hence, many disabled and nondisabled are still like strangers with one another. This is understandable because when we lack knowledge, we tend to be uncomfortable about our own abilities. What would we say to someone with a disability? Perhaps we would do the wrong thing!

It does appear, however, that institutional care and special school settings are needed for some individuals. The degree of the disability may make such an arrangement the most appropriate. The important issue is to be sure that segregation and inappropriate placement are minimized.

Another factor affecting our perception of the disabled is advertising in the American culture. Television, radio, and other advertising emphasize having a "body beautiful." The theme of physical perfection is widespread. The discrepancy between the models we admire for physical attributes and what exists in most of us is greater for the disabled than the physically normal. Much of today's society still has problems in distinguishing "different" from "abnormal." Most of us realize that few physically normal individuals compare well with the beautiful models and handsome actors. Indeed, most of us have defects such as poor eyesight, overweight, hair loss, crooked teeth, or stringy hair, but some defects are more visible.

With recent efforts to expose the disabled and physically normal populations to one another, differences are becoming increasingly minimized. In time and with effort, it should be possible for us to see the *person* in the wheelchair rather than the wheelchair with the person in it. Disabled people are beginning to say, "Our bodies may make us disabled, but it is society which makes us handicapped." It is the willingness of the physically normal to change their perceptions and the disabled to fight for changes which gives us hope for an enlightened future.

Is Society Changing?

These are exciting times as people with disabilities begin to assert their rights. Together with concerned parents and professionals, they are pressing for "mainstreaming" or "normalization." These terms signify the move to bring people with disabilities into the mainstream of society so that they can live more normal lives.

There are three areas where mainstreaming is occurring. The first comes early in a child's life when school begins. New federal law now mandates that every child with a disability has the right to attend school in the "least restricted environment."

Secondly, the new rights of the disabled include accessibility to all public buildings which have utilized federal money for construction. Those operating privately funded buildings should recognize their moral responsibilities to make such changes. Oftentimes the building, not the disability, may be the barrier to a more normal life.

Thirdly, the disabled now have equal access to employment. Federal laws prohibit discrimination in hiring the disabled. Children with disabilities need to grow up knowing that they will be able to compete equally for jobs. Changes in these three areas have occurred rapidly in recent years, and more changes can be expected in the future. Changing attitudes is, however, a difficult task!

What Can You Do to Help?

Changes in society begin in your own home. You should encourage your child to participate in activities outside the house, attend public events, be active in school, play with neighborhood children, engage in regular or special recreational programs, and believe in himself and his abilities. In doing so, he will project the kind of image needed

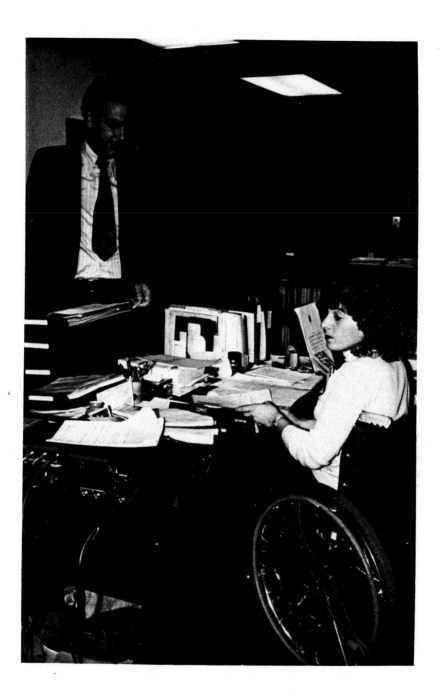

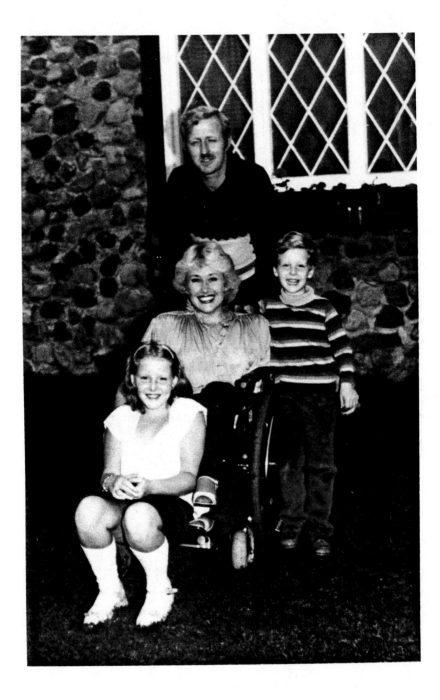

to make the disabled truly a part of the mainstream. If you have any energy left, look for political and social action groups for the disabled where your opinion can be magnified through group action to have the greatest impact.

CHAPTER 10

GROWING UP IN MIND AND BODY

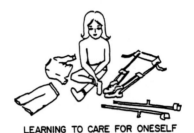

LEARNING TO CARE FOR ONESELF

Figure 10-1.

How Children Learn New Tasks

A USEFUL way to consider how children develop from infancy into adulthood is through a series of steps. Each step is a task which must be learned. The encouragement to move on from one step to another comes from a variety of sources. However, the following major areas are those most influential in determining how your child will develop.

(1) Cues from physical surroundings
(2) Challenges from playmates
(3) Expectations from parents
(4) Demands from school and society

These steps must be learned at a certain time and in a certain manner for development to be smooth and for children to keep up with their peers. Children who are unable to learn certain tasks will not only be restricted from becomming skilled in that particular area but may also be prevented from learning other tasks which come later. When this happens, children can remain at a certain level for a prolonged time. These delays may be mild and almost unnoticeable, or they may be very marked and require special treatments, programs, or services.

Some tasks which a child must learn are more important than others. In order to understand better how children with spina bifida develop, let us first consider what all children need to learn in each major developmental period. These periods are:

Infancy
Early childhood

64

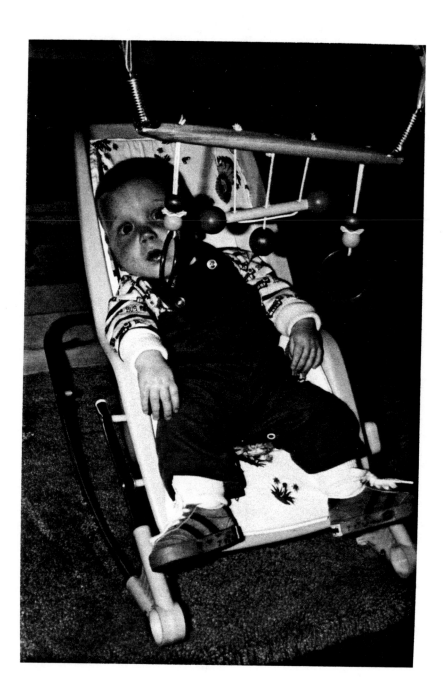

Middle childhood
Adolescence
Adulthood

Major Tasks to Be Learned by All Children
for Each Period of Development

Infancy (0-2 years)

(A) Begins to explore and learn about his environment by the use of vision, hearing, touch, taste, and feel.
(B) Starts to move around independently.
(C) Gains control over eating.
(D) Begins to communicate by use of sounds, words and gestures.
(E) Starts learning through trial and error.
(F) Starts to separate himself from the external world by developing ideas about space, time and what causes things to happen.
(G) Starts to identify specific people as important in his life.
(H) Develops a feeling of trust for important people in his life.
(I) Starts developing a personality unique to himself.

Early Childhood (2-5 years)

(A) Expands language use, particularly the ability to put together words into increasingly complex sentences, i.e. "go to store."
(B) Learns to obey basic rules given by parents and other adults. Obeying rules seem to result from a dawning awareness of the adult's authority and the bad consequences if they do not do what adults want. At this age children are not able to judge what is right or wrong, i.e. learn not to pull the dog's tail. Soon to come is the development of a conscience.
(C) Start to learn about social contact with other than immediate family.
(D) Begin to master small and large movements of the body in order to play children's games, move about independently, and start taking care of himself.
(E) Successfully meets a challenge and gains a sense of mastery. Parents urging him to perfect his skills at this time is crucial to preventing development of shame and doubt.
(F) Becomes aware of specific aspects of his physical development and forms attitudes about his own body.
(G) Recognizes that boys and girls are physically different from each other.
(H) Identifies with parents how they act and what they do.
(I) Through play activities with toys and games with peers, learns about his capabilities and begins to handle stress.

In spite of all these tasks that children must learn, the understanding of preschool children is still very simple and self-centered. They tend to interpret things only from their own experience and viewpoint. This typically results in disagreements with playmates as well as parents.

Middle Childhood (5-12 years)

(A) Enters school without too much distress about leaving home.
(B) Gets along with friends and becomes a member of a small group for class or games.
(C) Learns the appropriate rules for different settings — such as the playground, home, school, church, stores, etc., i.e. taking turns on the playground and sitting quietly in church.
(D) Learns to coordinate several bits of information or viewpoints at the same time. This is shown in. the ability to group and classify objects and to make judgments. These can be practical or even moral judgments if the information is fairly obvious. These understandings are necessary to learning basic academic skills such as reading, writing, and arithmetic.
(E) Starts to think about solutions to problems rather than using trial and error.
(F) Comes to understand concepts of time and space, cause and effect, and quantities in a much more "adult manner."
(G) Personal and sexual identities are further developed through pressures and examples from parents, friends, and popular figures. Although every child is unique, children of this age want to conform in dress, behavior, likes and dislikes.

More than anything else, a school-age child is a doer. He is constantly active and absorbed in a variety of physical and intellectual activities. Only if his activities are rewarded with success will be begin to see himself as a competent doer. He does not have to succeed at everything, but only often enough to keep him motivated and continuing to try. During this age he comes to see himself as capable in certain areas, i.e. math, reading, and less capable in others, i.e. sports. As a result of these experiences he moves into adolescence with a definite feeling about himself and his abilities.

Adolescence (12-18 years)

(A) Experiences dramatic bodily growth and changes and accepts these as part of his new image.
(B) Gradual social and emotional separation from parents in an effort to become independent.
(C) Identifies future life interests or careers.
(D) Develops sex role which is acceptable by society. This eventually leads to preparation for marriage and other adult responsi-

bilities.

(E) Enjoys new privileges and comes to accept the responsibilities that go along with them.

(F) Participates in crushes and cliques. Comes to see himself as a more natural member of certain groups.

(G) Becomes capable of abstract and complex reasoning.

(H) Begins to develop a set of personal beliefs or values necessary for becoming a responsible citizen.

Adolescence is a time of mixed feelings for both parent and child. Both want independence to occur but have mixed feelings and fears in letting it happen.

Adulthood (18-years)

(A) Solidifies identity.

(B) Shares a mutual trust, generally with a selected member of the opposite sex.

(C) Achieves interdependence with others and a place in society.

(D) Completes job selection and career choice.

(E) Ready to take on responsibility for the welfare of others.

It should be noted that for most children, certain tasks, i.e. walking, are faced only once, whereas others, i.e. social behavior, may be faced repeatedly. Different stages require different social responses.

Promoting the Best Development in Your Child with Spina Bifida

The learning of the developmental tasks we have reviewed is taken for granted with most children. By contrast, many people automatically assume a disabled child will not be able to accomplish any tasks within a reasonable time. In fact, most of the usual tasks can be achieved by the child with spina bifida. They may be more challenging for both the child and the parent, but they can be accomplished. The following are some suggestions on how to accomplish them.

Emphasize the Positive

There will be many things which your child can do correctly and at the appropriate age. You can influence your child's developmental progress by responding positively to these behaviors. The following are some ways you can guide your child's behavior in the desired direction:

(1) Approve (reward) behaviors which are appropriate and which you want him to continue. Your child will tend to repeat them.

(2) Ignore (no reward) behaviors which are not appropriate and you would like him to stop. They will tend not to be repeated.

Parents should be aware of other affects their responses to various situations may cause. A *general* lack of attention or rewards for behavior can delay developmental progress. This lack of stimulation slows or prevents the learning of new skills. This sometimes is a problem when children are cared for in institutions. This general lack of stimulation is different than ignoring specific, inappropriate behaviors for the purpose of eliminating them. Such severe deprivation rarely occurs in families, but sometimes attention or stimulation is offered in only a limited or sporadic fashion. It is not clear if this delays development also, but it is best not to take chances. To avoid insufficient stimulation, you should develop a routine so your child can plan on certain activities and on receiving your attention during a certain time. This is a necessary first step before you can start to work on rewarding certain desired behaviors such as independence or good manners.

Choosing the best type of reward can make a great deal of difference in how your child responds. A popular way to reward children is to give them something *material* such as a toy. It is best not to use food as a reward since weight control is difficult in children with spina bifida. Generally material rewards are less effective than *social* rewards, such as consistent praise and attention when your child demonstrates the desired behavior.

Punishment for undesirable behavior has been found to be less effective than ignoring the incident entirely. Certain children get some reward out of the attention which comes from punishment itself, but when undesirable behavior is ignored the child finds it boring. Sooner or later, he will demonstrate the desirable behavior again. When this happens, consistent praise will make that behavior more interesting for him and more likely to be repeated.

Encourage Independence

The first step to independence is for your child to take an *active* rather than a passive role in his environment. Whenever possible, he should be encouraged to manipulate, explore and discover things on his own rather than simply being told or shown about them. A child comes to understand himself only after he has actively explored his environment.

Encouraging independence is particularly difficult for parents of a disabled child. Besides figuring out how physical limitations can affect his participation in various tasks, it is admittedly hard for parents to know if they are rewarding the correct behaviors. Despite the difficulties, this area deserves your attention and study. You can consciously or unconsciously maintain a child's helplessness and immaturity by rewarding dependent behaviors and not rewarding independent action.

AN EXAMPLE OF REWARDING INDEPENDENT BEHAVIOR: Mary is seven and has an ileal conduit which she has been trying to care for by herself. The first several times she tried to apply her appliance, she did not center the adhesive disc correctly around the stoma. Two hours later the entire appliance fell off creating a mess. This upset her greatly. She knew that when mother did the appliance it stayed on very well. Mary's mother was also upset and was tempted to apply the disc herself. Supplies were being wasted and a lot of time was being spent on this project. Instead mother offered encouragement to her daughter and described again how to center the adhesive disc properly. Mother selected a time when both of them were relaxed and could practice with the appliance. In doing so, mother made a long-term investment in Mary's eventual independence. The beginning days were time consuming and full of errors and frustration, but mother was counting on Mary becoming more skilled as time passed and her experience grew. More importantly, Mary saw her mother had confidence that she could learn this task. Her efforts were being positively rewarded by her mother's attitude. She was encouraged to continue practicing and will eventually achieve her goal.

AN EXAMPLE OF REWARDING DEPENDENT BEHAVIOR: John is eight years old. He is learning to put on his long leg braces in the morning before school. This task is one with which he struggles and takes a long time. His father would love for him to learn this chore, but he feels there is not enough time in the morning to let him practice. Father steps in and puts the braces on after John tries only a few minutes.

John learns to depend on Father's stepping in after a few minutes. He knows father will rescue him from the struggle. John has no encouragement to work faster or more efficiently and learn this skill. It is a relief to be momentarily rescued from this challenging situation, but John may never learn this task. Even worse, he may grow to feel that he is *unable* to accomplish this or even other tasks.

Father has made a short-term investment. John was on time for the school bus today, but Father may find himself putting on the braces for years to come. Father is frustrated and cannot understand why his son does not take more initiative or show more skill. John senses his father's feelings about him and does not feel very good about himself.

Promote Socialization

Paralysis of parts of your child's body or other physical or mental limitations can interfere with his experiencing a variety of *real life situations*. This lack of experience and exposure to various other people affects the area of development called socialization. How well socializing skills are developed influences how confident and flexible he will be in meeting the everyday challenges of life.

You can decrease the effects of these limitations by some of the following steps:

ENCOURAGE SMALL GROUP EXPERIENCES. Examples are nursery schools, neighborhood play groups or clubs. Participation in these groups can teach skills in communication, sharing and responsibility. They can also help broaden your child's viewpoint of himself and others.

BE SURE YOUR CHILD BECOMES MORE MOBILE (crawl, sit, stand, ambulate). This should happen for your child at approximately the same time as his friends (see mobility). Professional programs, such as nurseries with provisions for the disabled, can help you improve your child's coordination and maximize his use of any equipment.

BE CREATIVE. Sponsor activities around the house which might attract playmates. Any planned group can be a source of stimulation. You should avoid taking the place of your child attracting his own friends. If playmates are automatically available through someone else's efforts, he may not develop the pleasing personality traits which are needed to attract friends.

HELP HIM DEVELOP PERSONAL-SOCIAL SKILLS. Your child needs personal and social skills for dealing with others. He needs to recognize, accept and feel good about the skills he does have. There are several ingredients which help children become competent in these areas.

LIVING IN A PREDICTABLE, CONSISTENT ENVIRONMENT. If you want your child's behavior to be predictable, he must find you consistent and predictable in dealing with him. He needs consistent limits set on him and some sort of household routine. This ability will help him join in social groups more easily.

ALLOW OPPORTUNITIES FOR CHOICE OR RISK. Setting up situations in which your child can make decisions and take small chances is an important part of building a good feeling about himself. It is easy for parents or other adults to make decisions or do things for a disabled child without recognizing that it deprives him of participating in the activity. The types of choices and chances should be related to the age and needs of your child. They can range from simple choices, such as what to eat or wear, to more mature choices, such as what to do or where to spend leisure time.

Encouraging Sexual Development

This is an important area of development. Oftentimes people assume sexual issues do not pertain to the disabled, but this is not true. Generally this is because there is confusion about how the disabled will function sexually when they get older. You will need to encourage your child to develop a sense of maleness or femaleness.

You should recognize that disabled children are just as much a boy or girl (and eventually a man or woman) as any other child. They

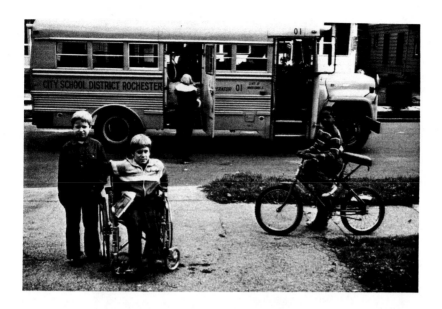

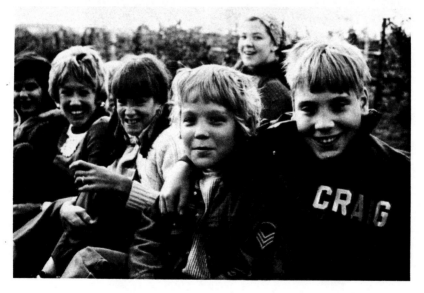

A Field Day.

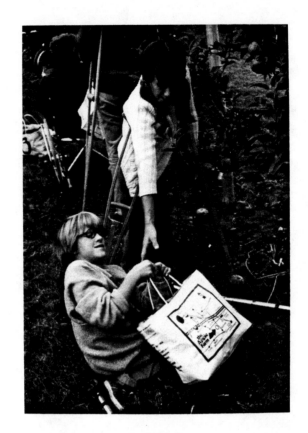

A Field Day.

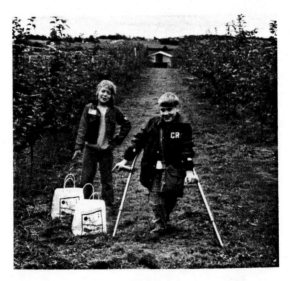

A Field Day.

need to be encouraged to pursue play activities and to dress in clothing appropriate for their sex. Today we tend toward less rigid definitions about what boys and girls can do, but there generally remain some traditional ideas about how each sex should act. Children with spina bifida have the same needs as other children for appropriate sex education. If you neglect this natural aspect of growing up, it conveys the message that sexuality-related issues are not relevant to them. The most effective models for sexual identity remain a boy's father and a girl's mother. Children will imitate their parents in this area as well as others. It will not be until the teen years that questions will become more technical and the "how to" of sexual functioning assumes importance. By that age, they will be able to understand the wide variety of ways in which the general population functions sexually.

Rules For Helping Your Child Develop

You should act in the manner you want your child to behave. Your behavior serves as a *model* for your child to follow.

Consistent *acceptance* of your child with *rewards* for his appropriate actions will encourage your child to repeat them.

Providing a *stimulating* environment will help your child accomplish the tasks appropriate for his age. Take into consideration his disability but challenge his skills.

Balance your efforts in different areas of his development so he will gain skills in all areas, i.e. intellectual, social, motor skills, etc.

Learn to *recognize* the skills your child possesses, so you can help him decide on realistic future goals and how to attain them.

YOUR CHILD'S EDUCATIONAL NEEDS

Children with spina bifida need an appropriate education to prepare them for a happy and productive life. For the physically disabled child, one important goal is making the most of intellectual potential and social abilities. For that reason, education for the child with a disability is not only a need, but a basic right. Knowledgeable parents have demanded this, and some state and local governments have responded through new laws guaranteeing the disabled equal rights to an education. Generally this has contributed to a more mainstreamed approach to education where disabled students are taking their place in classrooms with their physically normal peers. Although this may not be possible for every disabled student, more decisions are being made based on intellectual abilities rather than physical disabilities.

What Abilities Do Most Children with Spina Bifida Have?

Over two thirds of children with spina bifida have normal

intelligence when formal psychological testing is performed. This means their intelligence quotient (IQ) is within the normal range of 80 to 120. Many of them fall within the lower part of the normal range, a few are brighter than normal, and some are below the normal limits. The intellectual and social abilities of children with spina bifida are one of their most important assets, and when adequately developed permit some to compete with other adults in later life.

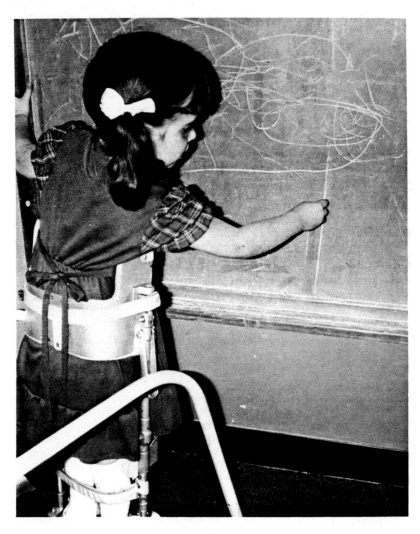

Figure 10-2.

What Special Needs Do Children with Spina Bifida Have?

Their special needs center around three areas: Learning, Social Skills, and Personal Care Skills.

LEARNING. Having intelligence generally within the normal range will be a tremendous asset for your child throughout life. Despite this, you need to be aware that your child may experience some of the special learning problems which occur in normal children. These learning disabilities are statistically more prevalent in the spina bifida group and include problems with hand-eye coordination and visual perception, among other things. A special evaluation for the presence of learning disabilities early in your child's school career may be beneficial.

SOCIAL SKILLS. Your child has the same needs as does every child to socialize and interact with peers of all sizes, shapes and backgrounds. Opportunities to do so occur less frequently, however, for the child who has problems with mobility. You will need to make special efforts to insure he engages in normal activities for his age both at school and at home.

PERSONAL CARE SKILLS. All children need to progress through various stages of learning to care for themselves. Your child is no exception to this rule. You should work at home right from the beginning to teach him self-care at approximately the same time as other children. Accomplishing these goals will be more difficult for your child. You would be wise to see that his self care efforts continue while he is at school also. It may be possible to set up a program where he can continue working on those tasks under the supervision (be sure they do not perform the task for him) of selected school staff. Be sure this does not detract too much from learning time for academic subjects, and be realistic about what you expect the school staff to accomplish.

Planning for Your Child's Education

Planning for your child's education requires careful consideration of his special needs. The following are some questions for which you will need some answers:

1. Is there adequate transportation to the school?
2. Will the child need assistance getting in and out of a vehicle?
3. Is the school building accessible?
4. Is the school physically arranged so that he can participate in physical education, art or music class, lunch room, or field trips?
5. Are toilet facilities adequate and will he have privacy?
6. Is toileting assistance available?
7. Is there a school nurse or other staff available for physical care

and emotional support?

8. Can physical therapy be made available if necessary?

There may be so much energy devoted to planning for these physical problems that parents and school officials lose sight of planning for the child's learning. Because of the significant number of learning disabilities experienced by children with spina bifida, your child may benefit from extra classroom help in certain areas. You may need to find the answers to the following questions early in the educational program:

1. Does the instructional (academic) program meet his needs and his abilities?
2. Is a "resource room" available to supplement a regular classroom?
3. Will the child do better in a part-time or full-time special class, where instruction could concentrate on specific learning needs?

Some Problems in Obtaining an Adequate Education

It is in your child's best interests if the school district, the parents and your health care providers work together to develop the most appropriate program. For some families, this experience is enlightening and reassuring. For others, it is tedious and frustrating.

Until recently, disabled children were often denied admission to public schools because they did not "fit in." Today the situation is improved by laws which provide some type of educational services for disabled children in each of the fifty states. Recent court decisions and federal legislation (Public Law 94-142) have mandated the right of disabled children to have a public education. However, parents still encounter problems in achieving this. Occasionally, children are still being excluded from a full school program with excuses such as he "lacks toilet training" or "his condition is too delicate."

Parents may encounter difficulties with school districts that are unwilling or unable to provide needed services. Transportation, for example, is an essential service to which children with spina bifida are entitled, but you may find it difficult to obtain. Parents should be aware of local education laws regarding their school districts' responsibility for such services. These laws are sometimes vague. For example, in 1976 New York State mandated that local school districts provide transportation for disabled children in special classes. The school districts' responsibility to mainstreaming these children in regular classes was less clear. If local school officials cannot clarify such issues or you have difficulty in obtaining services, an appeal to the State Commission of Education, an attorney's opinion, or a petition to a family court are other methods you should consider.

What Parents Can Do to Help

INFORM YOUR SCHOOL SYSTEM. Parents can alleviate fears and promote cooperation with school systems by making sure that administrators, teachers and school health staff are fully aware of their child's disability, abilities and activity level. Any medication your child receives should be a part of the school file. You should personally explain health problems to the school staff who have contact with your child. School personnel may have unnecessary anxieties about possibly harming your child by allowing him to fully participate in school activities. You should convey your own attitudes about promoting independence and risk taking to those at school. Speaking to school personnel can encourage them to have a more positive view of your child's abilities.

Children with spina bifida often need personal care assistance in school. School districts are often cooperative in providing help from an aide or school nurse, but difficulties can arise. Some parents find they must offer to visit the school and either help or demonstrate how procedures are done before the school district agrees to be responsible. Such parent involvement can be especially helpful in relieving the anxiety of the school staff. An important ally in this particular situation is a school nurse, if one is available. Contact with the nurse before the onset of the school year will place her in a better position to help your child when school begins. If those at school do not understand your child's special needs, they may become very anxious. Besides helping with your child's physical needs, the nurse is responsible for interpreting his physical needs and programs to the rest of the school staff throughout the year. In order to do so, the nurse should be informed about the following:

1. Spina bifida as it pertains to your child's special case (shunt, ileal loop, degree of paralysis, ambulation equipment, etc.)
2. Your child's abilities and areas where assistance will be needed (self-catheterization, bowel program, dressing self, change ileal loop equipment, etc.).
3. Medication requirement.
4. Immunizations and results of physical examinations.

Learn How the Education System Works

As parents of a child with special needs, you need to learn how your state and local education systems work. This knowledge can relieve some of your anxiety about how decisions are made for your child's education. It will also allow you to effectively work for your child's best interests. Opportunities vary in districts and states. To illustrate, the following is a short description of how educational placement of disabled children is determined in New York State.

It is the responsibility of the local school district to determine the educational needs of the child and place him in the most appropriate program based on these needs. By state law, each school district is required to have a Committee on the Handicapped which identifies, reviews, and evaluates the status of each disabled child in their district at least once a year. The law also requires that parents be informed when their child is reviewed by this group. Parents should be aware that if the recommended placement is not acceptable to them, they may appeal to the Board of Education for an impartial hearing. It is now required that school districts develop individual educational plans for each child. Parents must be included in this planning. As a general matter of policy, parents should confer regularly (usually at the time of report cards) with the teacher and other school staff. They should discuss the child's progress, school placement, needs and plans for the future.

The Committee on the Handicapped in each school district must include a psychologist, a teacher or administrator of special education, a physician, a parent of a handicapped child residing in that school district, and other individuals at the district's discretion. Individual psychological testing is an essential service that schools should provide to assure recognition of possible learning problems and insure proper school placement and services. New York State requires initial psychological testing, and also retesting, of disabled children in special programs at least once every three years.

Know the Types of School Programs

Parents should know what educational programs and alternatives are available in their community. It is even more important that they be aware of the most appropriate program to best meet the individual needs of their child. It is a good idea for parents to select a program that allows a maximum amount of contact with nondisabled pupils, and one that is near your neighborhood and meets your child's physical, learning and social needs.

School program alternatives may be limited in some communities, but the following will give you an idea of the levels of programs which are *ideally* available in each district.

Program	*Description*
1. Preschool and preventive program.	District-wide program with emphasis on family guidance and counseling along with development of learning, emotional and physical skills in all pupils.
2. Regular class	Children not in need of academic sup-

	portive services. May have supportive services for personal care.
3. Regular class with academic supportive services	Children would continue in regular class with extra supportive services, such as psychological, social, and speech-language therapy. Nursing and physical therapy support would be available if needed.
4. Regular class with supplementary instructional services	Assignment of special itinerant teachers for remedial reading, speech-language, learning disabilities, etc.
5. Part-time special resource class	Part-time attendance in regular programs and part-time with a special education resource teacher or special educational class for specific instruction in specific areas of need.
6. Special education class with integration for special subjects	Attendance in special education class for "academics" but included with regular class pupils for special subjects, i.e. physical education, music, art.
7. Full-time special education class	Attendance in special education class with supportive instruction and services for personal care.
8. Home-hospital instruction	Temporary individual or small group tutoring at home or in a hospital setting during convalescence.

Mainstreaming

Although it is desirable that the special needs of a child be met, it is usually preferable that a child attend a program which is as similar to the regular class program as possible. Gradually students should progress towards regular programs as long as their special needs are being met. Such mainstreaming enriches the lives of all children. It also provides experiences that will encourage understandings and tolerances between those who are disabled and those who are not in our future society.

Educational Needs at Different Ages

The Importance of Preschool Education

Preparation for your child's education should begin early, probably earlier than you are anticipating. Ideally, your child should enter school ready to learn what is being taught, able to mix socially with other children and feeling fairly good about himself. The successful development of these abilities occurs in preschool years. Children with disabilities such as spina bifida especially benefit from opportunities for early socialization and independence. Such experiences improve their self-awareness and lessen the chance of developing or continuing handicapping behavior. The early recognition of delayed learning skills will also allow for better planning of additional services when the child enters school.

Age 2 to 3 Years

At this age most children are becoming more independent and rapidly developing social skills. A program of socialization and stimulation is especially important at this age for the child with spina bifida. It will help offset the periods of confinement due to hospitalization or immobility at home. Organized community programs are often available for children with physical disabilities. Check with local agencies that deal with disabled children, or contact your local Community Chest. Another consideration is a day care program for normal children. They may accept your child. If no organized program exists, you may want to consider developing one yourself.

Age 3 Years

Continued exposure to other children and the acquisition of new skills are important goals this year. Nursery schools or other organized programs should be investigated. By the end of this year, you should have a better awareness of your child's abilities and the areas in which he needs special help.

You should make contact with the school district at this time. Make an appointment to meet with the Pupil Personnel Director, the Principal, or the chairman of the local committee which recommends school placement for children with disabilities. Discuss the placement of children with spina bifida who are already being educated. Bring up some of the issues presented in "Planning for your Child's Education." Are efforts at mainstreaming likely to be strengthened in the next four years? How does the school district want you to cooperate with them during the preschool years?

Age 4 Years

The preschool program this year should be directed toward helping your child in areas which need special attention. Selected learning skills, social skills or independence training are the major areas. Some of these skills can be strengthened with continued help, but others may need to be accepted as what your child is able to achieve.

Parents should now begin discussing the specifics of their child's educational placement within the school district. The pupil services director should be able to identify which school your child will attend and what services he will have available. You should meet with the principal of that school and, if possible, the teacher and school nurse. This will allow you to explain your child's physical and emotional condition, answer questions, and convey attitudes regarding your child's needs and abilities. You should have a picture of a typical day in school for your child. Then you can explain to him what the school will expect. This mutual sharing of knowledge and expectations will reduce anxieties and help both the school and your child to accomplish the desired educational goals.

Kindergarten (Age 5 Years)

If your school district does not have a preschool program for your child, this will be the first school experience for him. You, as well as your school district, will want your child to be in a program that will encourage learning. It is your school district's responsibility, mandated by law, to offer an appropriate program for children at this age. The program should help him:

- develop a desire to learn
- develop a positive self-image
- learn to work and play well with others
- grow in a learning setting that promotes and protects health and well-being
- learn that the world has an "order" and "routine" that can be understood and managed at his individual level of development
- become more independent and self-directive

The school district's Committee on the Handicapped is responsible for reviewing your child's status and determining the most appropriate school and/or program placement. This decision is based on individual needs. (See "How the Education System Works") You are entitled to know and should be informed of the:

- recommended placement
- proposed classification and reasons why this classification was deemed appropriate
- tests or reports used
- availability of records for their review and interpretation
- right to obtain a hearing if you have objections to the committee's recommendations
- procedures of appeal
- opportunities for independent educational evaluation

Good communication on a regular basis between you and the school personnel is essential, and should include a progress report and a discussion of your child's needs. The teacher, in particular, needs to understand how health and emotional factors may influence learning.

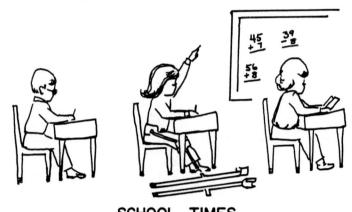

SCHOOL TIMES

Figure 10-3.

Primary School (Grades 1-3, Ages 5-8)

During the primary grades your child will attend an elementary school. It is the responsibility of your school district to offer an appropriate educational program beginning with the first grade. During the primary school years, your child should be introduced to and develop the following:

- Skills in basic vocabulary, language, reading, and arithmetic.
- Skills in locating and discussing information.
- An understanding of the physical and social environment through social studies, science and the arts.
- An inquiring mind.
- An ability to think independently and cooperatively.

Teachers will periodically measure your child's individual growth and development, particularly in reading and arithmetic. Some children will need, and should receive, additional remedial assistance. This may be done by the classroom teacher, reading teacher, speech and language teacher, psychologist, social worker, or others.

Middle School (Grades 4-6, Ages 9-11)

These grades are considered the intermediate years in the elementary school program. During these years, the general goals of the instructional program should include:

- continuing the development of basic reading, language and mathematics skills.
- applying these basic skills through inquiry into the content areas

of social studies, science and the arts.

- developing research skills and techniques.
- broadening awareness of career opportunities.
- developing an understanding and use of decision-making processes.
- providing opportunities for self-expression through pursuit of individual talents and interests.

Junior High School (Grades 7-8, Ages 12-13)

As your child enters the junior or junior-senior high school, there is an adolescent search for self-identification. It is common for students at this level to be intently trying to answer the question, "Who am I?" During this search, the child often moves away from the family and closer to peer groups. These are the developmental years during which the adolescent is moving towards increasing independence in all phases of his life.

The transition from the elementary school to the junior high is an important and major one. You should be sure that the junior high school has the proper information regarding your child's academic, physical and behavioral functioning. This is best done by having a junior high school counselor from the school to which your child is assigned visit the elementary school and confer with his teachers. The Committee on the Handicapped should continue to review your child's placement yearly and they should furnish the new school staff with information and recommendations.

You should get to know the school counselor, since he can be a "key" person in the high school setting. Counselors help with educational and vocational planning, program changes, and personal problems. They also assist in identifying interests, strengths, and limitations. They can help your child plan and work toward future goals, whether those be further education or an occupation. They should meet regularly with you and your child.

The role of the school nurse should be similar to that in the earlier grades, and the nurse may become more involved in health and self-care teaching now that your child is older and more capable.

Senior High School (Grades 9-12, Ages 14-17)

Your high school should provide a program in line with your child's physical and intellectual capabilities. The counselor, parents, and student should outline a total grade 9-12 course plan. This is the best way to help meet the district's graduation requirements prior to completion of the twelfth grade.

Most parents hope their child has some planned direction for his life prior to completion of high school, but this is not always the case.

Your child may need special help in preparing for the future. A high school counselor should be readily available and can help in selecting an educational program that prepares him for the future. Psychological, educational, achievement and interest evaluations may be needed to help formulate an appropriate educational plan. Periodic conferences with either the school counselor and/or the pupil service team (school psychologist, social worker, nurse) may be helpful.

During the ninth grade, you should contact the local Office of Vocational Rehabilitation. Habilitation assistance, such as further education or job training and preparation, may be available. This service is often available to anyone in the community who has a health or physical problem severe enough to prevent their finding employment, further their education or training through normal channels. Early contact with a Vocational Rehabilitation agency will give them more time to develop a plan for your child.

Does Spina Bifida Affect a Child's Intelligence?

The majority of children with spina bifida have intelligence within the normal range. Despite that reassuring fact, most parents fear their infant will be mentally retarded in addition to having a physical disability. This fear is understandable in view of the early attention focused on the infant's head size, the involvement of the nervous system, and everyone's concern about the child and his future.

The following information may give you a better perspective on this issue. Two-thirds of children with spina bifida score within the average range on intelligence tests. Although intelligence scores are probably overrated in their ability to predict how well a child will do in school, they do offer a method of comparing the intelligence ability of one child with another. Intelligence scores (I.Q.) in the range of 80 to 120 are considered average in the sense that most people score within this range. Many children with spina bifida do fall in the lower part of the range, but are still within the normal limits. Children with spina bifida who fall below this average range are usually not far below. Despite these abilities, many children with spina bifida have a difficult time learning. These learning disabilities have many causes and can be helped if properly recognized and handled.

Are Intelligence Evaluations Always Accurate?

Those involved in evaluating children say it is difficult to predict a young child's intelligence. As a child gets older the results of intelligence evaluations become more reliable, because he is better able to show his skills. Tests, of course, have limitations and a single score may be misleading. Everyone has a bad day occasionally which can affect evaluation results. A temporary physical illness, unfamiliarity with surroundings, or a special sight or hearing problem could also interfere. Should you feel this is the case with your child, bring your thoughts to the attention of the evaluator. Even so, as a parent you have the right to discuss the results of any testing with the person who evaluated your child if you wish to do so. The reliability of testing increases if on more than one occasion the results are similar.

A child may be quite capable in certain areas but deficient in others. Children who are in the low average range or fall below the normal range can still benefit from a carefully designed educational program.

Learning about your child's intellectual skills, no matter what they are, can be an anxious event for you. The faster you can reach a realistic understanding of your child's intellectual capabilities the better. Most children are more comfortable when their abilities appropriately match what everyone is expecting of them.

A Child May Seem Brighter Than Testing Indicates

Children with hydrocephalus often communicate well with words. They may have good vocabularies and delight in social chatter. Those whose evaluation results indicate low or below average intelligence may seem to be brighter to parents and others because of this verbal ability. However, these talkative children often have problems when asked to use the words and thoughts in a meaningful way. The content of a child's speech and thoughts is what an intelligence test evaluates. Special psychologic, speech and language testing is sometimes useful in identifying more specific problem areas.

What Influences Intelligence

Children who have not needed shunts generally have intelligence scores similar to normal children. However, children with shunts more often score in the lower range of average intelligence compared to normal children. When children with spina bifida are compared to their normal brothers and sisters, they generally have a slightly lower IQ.

Shunts which need to be repaired for poor functioning or other reasons do not seem to lower the intelligence score. However, it is possible that damage could occur if the child is severely ill or has an episode where he receives inadequate oxygen. Infections in the shunt do seem to have an adverse effect and may lower intelligence scores.

Be Alert for Learning Problems

Many children with spina bifida have difficulties in learning

(learning disability) even though they have an average intelligence score. The exact reasons for this are not clear, but the following factors are thought to be related:

(1) overall intelligence
(2) perceptual motor problems
(3) emotional and social adjustment
(4) interest in learning
(5) school attendance
(6) adequacy of school program

Overall Intelligence

Most intelligence tests have two major components. One involves verbal abilities while the other looks at performance. Verbal skills include such subtests as comparing items, providing information about objects or topics, doing arithmetic, and explaining vocabulary words. Performance abilities are tasks like completing a picture which is missing a part, placing blocks in specific designs and putting puzzles together. Scores on both groups of subtests are then combined to arrive at an overall IQ score. If a child is very good in one area and very poor in another, the overall result would be average. This is what occurs in the presence of certain learning disabilities.

Emotional and Social Adjustment

Understanding and accepting ourselves and developing confidence in our abilities is an important step in growing up emotionally. A child's concept of himself is greatly influenced by the attitudes of those around him such as parents, brothers, sisters, relatives, friends, teachers, etc. If they feel the child will fail or cannot do a task, then the chances are good he will be unable to do it. Similarly, if expectations are positive and realistic, then even if the child fails initially, he will learn a little and be willing to try again. Having self-confidence and being willing to try are important parts of learning.

Interest in Learning

A desire to learn is also important. All children are able to learn best when they are interested in the topic or have some incentive to learn the material. This interest in learning results from the attitudes of the people around the child and their expectations of him. Successful learning is a good stimulus to learn more, and everyone needs positive experiences to keep his interest high. This makes it especially important that children with learning disabilities have their specific areas of competence identified early. Expectations from teachers and others must be realistic and within the child's abilities.

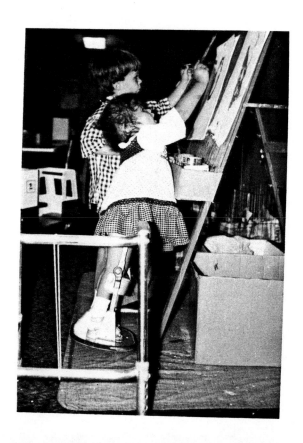

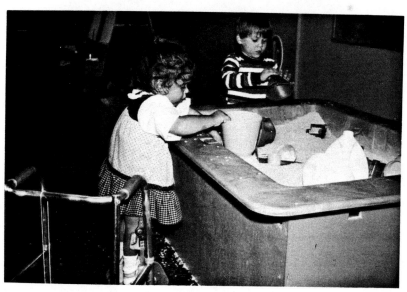

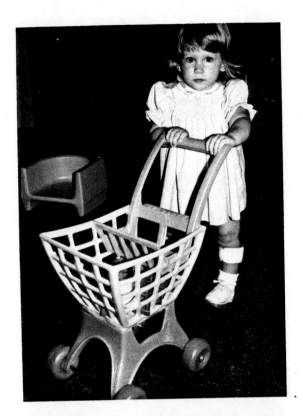

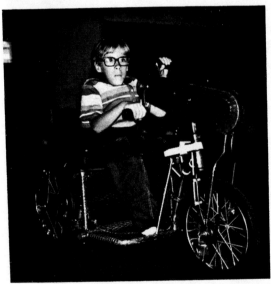

Hand-powered tricycle for children with paraplegia.

School Attendance

Children with spina bifida often have medical appointments or require hospitalization. This means that they cannot attend school classes at those times and, consequently, have interruptions in their learning and studying. It is more difficult to learn material and keep up with others in the class when school attendance is not regular.

Adequacy of School Program

A school program that is tailored to the individual child is very important. The program should focus on the child's abilities. It should provide successes so he will want to continue, and also help him improve in his weaker areas. It should meet his needs for interaction with other children and help him to improve his self-image by encouraging active participation in all aspects of school. This includes a physical education program adapted to his needs, rather than excluding him from the class.

Perceptual Motor Problem

Many children with spina bifida, especially those with shunts, have perceptual motor problems. These children may have difficulty separating figures from their background, identifying the difference between two similar letters, or coordinating their hands to thread beads, use scissors, or draw neatly. The child may have trouble recognizing differences between shapes or in coordinating the hands to do what the mind wants. Such perceptual problems or other factors affecting learning may explain why some children with spina bifida have difficulty in reading, writing, spelling and arithmetic.

Intellectual and Educational Needs

There is a wide range of intelligence levels and learning needs in normal children. The range in children with spina bifida is even broader. Learning and perceptual problems can be helped by a preschool readiness program or special help in school. The hope for all children is the best possible education; but for the child with spina bifida, this goal is even more important. A good education can compensate for some physical disabilities and help him prepare for a productive and happy life. Individual testing is necessary to help parents and educators plan the best possible school program and to identify those intellectual strengths which can be maximized and those weaknesses which can be either helped or must be accepted. Realistic goals and expectations will help your child reach his maximum capability.

RECREATION FOR YOUR CHILD

Recreation refers to the process of refreshing the body or mind by some form of play or amusement. The child with spina bifida needs the same opportunity for recreational activities as other children. After strenuous sessions, such as in physical therapy, your child may be even more in need of recreation. Fortunately, your child can enjoy and benefit from most of the "fun" types of play and hobbies. There are a few exceptions in certain forms of very physical recreation.

Playing with Your Infant

Infants with spina bifida derive the same satisfaction from playing with parents as do other infants. Holding, talking and laughing, playing peek-a-boo and other such activities are good recreation for both you and the baby. Between birth and one year of age such toys as mobiles, blocks and busy boxes are helpful.

Exploration of the environment is important to every young child. As soon as he is able to move around, whether it be by rolling himself from place to place, crawling or walking, a whole new world is opened for his pleasure. The physically disabled youngster may need special assistance to increase his mobility.

Several innovative toys are available for the crawling stage. A scooter board or "crawl-a-gator" may be useful at this stage. The child who is unable to crawl can be placed on the board. He lies on his stomach and by using his arms can learn to push himself along the floor. A caster cart is also hand operated. The young child can be in a sitting position, and maneuver it about by pushing on the wheels.

Around the ages of three to five years, your child is learning to socialize. Enrollment in a nursery school is a good beginning. Nursery school can also introduce him to arts and crafts activities and provide fun and relaxation along with the chance to improve coordination and dexterity. During the nursery school years, the teacher may identify areas of difficulty so help can be provided early. Successes in nursery school can also help foster a positive attitude. Trips to the park, zoo, circus or other events are exciting to any child.

By the age of three years, children become interested in exploring outside the home. Moving about on the sidewalk or around the yard presents special problems for the child with limited mobility. A recreational vehicle for this activity needs to be hand propelled, close to the ground, easily maneuverable, and fairly stable so it will not tip easily. Innovative toys such as the Krazy Car™ and Wild Rider™ (Marx Toy Company) are reasonably priced and meet these criteria. They can support and carry children up to 55 pounds in weight and maintain the interest of a child for many years. Hand-operated tricycles

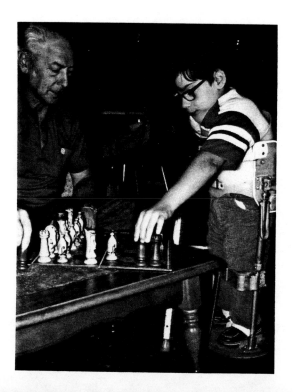

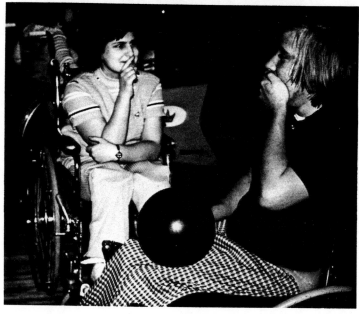

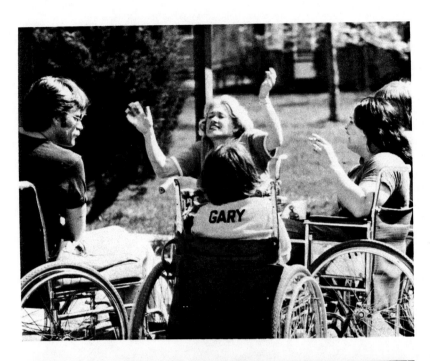

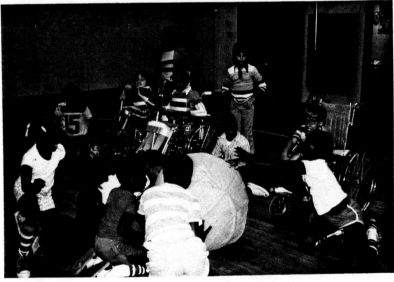

specially designed for children with paraplegia are just now becoming available on the market. Such tricycles can be useful for mobility in a neighborhood setting or for short distance transportation.

At age five or six years, children begin the formal school years. Emphasis is now placed on intellectual development. The school needs to recognize your child's abilities as well as his limitations. Special ramps, other equipment or facility changes may well be necessary to allow your child to move around independently and play with other children. Your child should be made to feel a part of the social life of the school as well as the academic part. It is important that interaction with other students be encouraged and that he receive neither excess attention nor special favors. Children need to learn how to compete fairly within their age group.

Inclusion in the physical education program is necessary in order to foster appropriate physical development. It can provide an opportunity to participate in organized games, and other activities. This recreational experience in the school relieves your child of some of the pressures resulting from the demands of structured academic activities. Children need this chance during the school day to relax and "blow off steam."

Extra-curricular activities at school such as special interest clubs and social clubs offer a good chance for social development. Clubs such as Boy and Girl Scouts and 4-H also help teach responsibility. Church groups and local community centers are other sources of these experiences.

Older children often become interested in making models, reading, musical instruments, working with electrical equipment, sewing, crafts and board games. These special interests should be encouraged. They offer your child the opportunity to participate on a par with children who are not disabled.

The stimulation of competitive sports for older children has been found to be a source of great self-accomplishment and pride. Larger metropolitan areas often have sports and athletic teams for the disabled such as in bowling, basketball and swimming. In some sports, such as pistol shooting and archery, disabled competitors can directly compete with others. Group activities such as these are particularly valuable in the teen years. The social benefits of the competition may be as great as the exercise and feeling of achievement. Often the interaction during competition helps the teens to become acquainted socially.

The culmination of athletic prowess for older teenagers with a disability is the International Paralympics. These precede the Olympics and are held every four years and in the same host country. In the paralympics, each country sends their disabled athletes who have previously qualified in such events as swimming, archery, fencing,

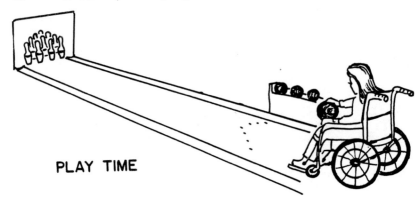

PLAY TIME

Figure 10-4.

weight lifting, basketball, track and field, etc. Competitors are individually evaluated and their degree of disability is matched. The competitors are true athletes and medals are awarded just as in the Olympics.

Recreation and athletics offer the disabled child the same rewards of relaxation and accomplishment open to other children. Parents of disabled children at times find it difficult to provide these opportunities, but they are probably a significant factor in growing up successfully.

SEX AND SEXUALITY

In order to discuss sexual issues we first need to understand the words to be used. *Sex* is a word used in many ways today. It can refer to whether one is male or female as well as the act of sex. *Sexuality* is a better term to describe many of the aspects related to sex. Sexuality means much more than the physical act. It includes how we and others view ourselves as males or females.

One builds views of oneself as a man or woman over many years. Early in childhood we begin to follow examples given by our mother, father and other significant people. This process of identifying with others of the same gender is part of sexuality. As we grow, the way we view ourselves is affected by the way other people respond to us as a male or female, or as a person in general. A girl who receives praise for her cooking may feel that being a good cook is the correct role to develop as a woman. A boy whose father thinks football is important may consider sports an important part of being a man. Our femininity or masculinity depends a great deal on the world around us.

Today's society allows people more freedom in expressing themselves in all aspects of their sexuality. Both men and women are being permitted to define their roles as they see fit. When people are comfortable with their sexuality, acknowledging a variety of approaches to the physical aspects of sex becomes easier and more acceptable. Sexual functioning with actual physical involvement between people is only one small part of a person's sexuality. Although sexuality and sex affect each other, they are not the same.

The Family Role in Sexuality

Our sexuality reflects an accumulation of our cultural experiences. We react to the clues we receive from our peers, family and society. For children with a physical disability, the world sometimes reacts first and strongest to differences in physical appearance. These children may find it difficult to obtain the same response from society as do the nondisabled children. In order to compensate, the family of a child with spina bifida may need to concentrate more than usual on reinforcing his postitive aspects. This will help him to develop a good self-image.

Despite the occasional special needs of children with spina bifida, you should encourage your child to be independent in self-care so that he can feel as good as possible about himself. He needs to be granted privacy, especially as the teenage years approach. Special attention may need to be given at this time to educating him about the opposite sex, since opportunities to gain personal experience may be fewer for the disabled child due to limited mobility.

Some of the difficulties in moving about hinder your child from relating to other teenagers. You can help by promoting as much independence as possible, so that he can learn social skills and develop his own private relationships. Occasionally street language and teenage slang terms may describe body feelings which your child lacks the sensation or experience to understand. If asked, you should help your teenager interpret some of these terms. As children with spina bifida grow to adulthood they need understanding, communication and factual information about their sexual capabilities. They deserve the same honest discussion about sex and sexuality as about other aspects of their disability. If your child has not raised this topic by the early teenage years, the discussion should be initiated by a family member. This is sometimes difficult for a parent to do, but children with disabilities deserve relief from this concern.

In this section we have provided only the general facts about sexual functioning in children with spina bifida. The details and degree of function a child has varies with each individual. The professionals caring for your child can help you understand his functioning before you begin any discussion with him.

The Male with Spina Bifida

Let us first discuss how spina bifida may affect male sexual functioning. Most of the medical information comes from working with males who have had a spinal cord injury rather than a birth defect. Even so, this can help our understanding of children with spina bifida, but there are some differences.

For males the nerves required to have an erection and ejaculation come from the lowest part of the spine. Almost all spina bifida lesions involve these nerves at least partially. The amount of damage to these nerves is quite variable, and only some of them may be involved. Therefore, for males sexual funcitoning can vary greatly between individuals, even when their spina bifida lesion is at the same level.

Many males have erections during bathing and self-care. Local skin contact can lead to an erection, even though this sensation may not be recognized or felt by the individual. The male with spina bifida may find this a helpful way of achieving an erection. There is also a decreased likelihood that "thoughts" alone will cause an erection.

The damage to the nerves of the lower spine can cause problems with ejaculation in those males where ejaculation can occur. The sperm may pass backwards into the bladder rather than leaving the end of the penis. As a result, only a small amount of fluid may pass outside, and the male with spina bifida may have difficulty fertilizing his partner. You should discuss your child's degree of paralysis and function with his physicians before you assume that he has or does not have some physical ability. Your child's personal experience, however, is the best barometer of what he is able to accomplish.

It is important to keep these issues in perspective. Lack of fertility should not be confused with diminished pleasure during sexual relations. Infertility is a problem which is shared by the population who are physically normal, as are other differences in sexual functioning. What is required by all partners, whether they are physically normal or disabled, is a willingness to modify techniques when needed. Just as various techniques have been developed over the years to optimize sexual pleasure among those without disabilities, so have they been developed among those with paraplegia or other less severe nerve damage. Exploration and experimentation is the place where any couple should begin in order to discover what is mutually enjoyable.

The Female with Spina Bifida

Females with spina bifida do not have the same concerns as males. Their female internal organs function in the same way as in other women. Some females with spina bifida have breast development and other adult sexual features earlier than their friends. Physical development may begin one to two years earlier, or occasionally as early as age six or seven years. Menstruation is similar to other females once it starts.

Fertility is normal, and child bearing is possible because the internal sexual organs are generally unaffected by the spina bifida. Women with spina bifida need regular gynecological examinations. They also need some type of birth control if they wish to avoid pregnancy when they are sexually active. During pregnancy the female with spina bifida needs careful medical supervision, since she may have more urine infections at that time. The birth canal should be checked to be sure it is large enough to allow for a vaginal delivery.

For some women with spina bifida, lack of sensation in the genital area results in the development of an accentuated sexual response from stimulating other parts of the body, such as the breasts. This is a type of compensation. Some positions during sexual relations are easier for a paralyzed female. If there is deceased genital skin sensation, her partner will need to help her avoid abrasions since she cannot protect herself. Care in providing lubrication, since this may not be adequate, can prevent problems. Women with spina bifida, like men, should feel free to explore various options for sexual expression with their partner. The goal is mutual pleasure in ways that are comfortable for both partners.

Issues Related to Sexual Intercourse

For those with spina bifida, there are other issues with which to deal during sexual intercourse. Avoiding leakage of urine is important, and patients with incontinence usually empty the bowel and bladder before beginning sexual relations. Even if there is an indwelling catheter, there are ways to manage this. Advance preparation is often the key to success.

Children with spina bifida sometimes have the urine diverted through an ileal loop. Occasionally teens will think that this also changes the location of sexual intercourse or functioning. This is not true and it should be made clear when the opportunity arises.

Those with paralysis occasionally experience severe headaches during sexual intercourse. This seems to result when stimulation of the genitals causes a rapid increase in blood pressure and then a headache. A brief pause during intercourse may relieve this if it is a problem. If this is a recurring problem, a physician can offer further help.

Other Sexual Options

All adults, but especially those disabled, need to explore other options and define their sexual functions more individually. Those with paralysis, like others, need to feel that this is a private, personal experience not to be judged by others. For many paralyzed people, experimentation and exploration with different techniques enables satisfying experiences and relationships. Books are available to aid the paralyzed person in understanding these options. (See Appendix A)

Learning to Communicate

For all of us, communication is an important part of any physical and emotional relationship. Expectations and the results of performance need to be discussed by couples. The physical concerns of one partner may become exaggerated unless they are openly shared with the other. Communication with your partner needs to occur on many levels (verbally, by touch, facial expression, etc.)

We all take risks when we communicate with another person. This is an especially risky venture to your personal image when it concerns sexual intimacy. Although communication in this area is difficult, the rewards are great. Some people discover they lack skills in communication and, therefore, have a difficult time developing a close relationship. This is a common problem which is not confined to those with spina bifida. You should realize that counseling is available to help people to be more at ease in thinking and talking about their feelings. To take advantage of these opportunities does not imply one is lacking, but only that one wants to be able to experience deeper and richer relationships with others.

When a relationship is between two people who care for each other, then satisfying sexual relations can become one part of this experience. All people need to sort out the extent to which sexual relations, love, reproduction and marriage are important to them. Then they can seek fulfillment in the various aspects with hopefully appropriate expectations.

CHILDREN'S CONCEPTS OF DEATH

Death is a painful subject and seems almost at odds with the rest of this book which discusses repair, restoration, and coping with a physical defect in such a way that your child can be integrated into your family and community as normally as possible. However, to neglect this issue would be a disservice to you, your family, and, particularly, your special child. It is for your family and those close to you that this chapter will be especially meaningful. It deals with a subject which has been occurring with less frequency in recent years to children with spina bifida, but death is still a greater threat to them than to the general population of children without a physical disability.

Fatal Complications of Spina Bifida

The highest incidence of death among children with spina bifida occurs during the first few days and weeks of life, when susceptibility to infection (especially meningitis) or complications from surgical repair are greatest. If no repair is undertaken, as in certain cases when the defect is very severe or when the child is not likely to tolerate surgery, there is a significant risk that meningitis will occur and may be fatal. Death can also occur from pneumonia, which is most frequently caused by the child's inability to clear mucus from air passages.

Beyond the newborn period, the two most common causes of death are shunt failure and progressive kidney damage. It is impossible to provide you with statistics about life expectancy. Reliable information is not available, because recent advances in treatment and habilitation have improved the prognosis of children with spina bifida dramatically during the past few years.

The risks described above are clearly not the usual ones exprienced by the average newborn. Despite these special challenges, *most* children with spina bifida do survive infancy and grow into adulthood. However, while growing up, your child may have occasion to worry about death. During periods of hospitalization, for example, your child or his siblings may fear that he will die. Parents can help ease these worries if they understand how children view death.

A Child's Understanding of Death

Although most descriptions of the development of the child's concept of death are based on chronological age, an individual child's concepts will be based on his own developmental level and his previous experiences. No two children are exactly alike. Some will seem very concerned or fascinated, while others will prefer not to mention or discuss serious illness or death. Your responses, in turn, will depend upon your degree of comfort with the topic, your own previous experiences, and the role religious beliefs play in your attitude toward death. Like children, no two adults are exactly alike either. However, parents and other involved family members, who may be called upon to answer questions or give comfort, should try to be consistent with the child. Thus, the answers he obtains from various people will be similar and, therefore, less confusing to him.

Understanding Death: 0-4 Years

Below the age of about four years, the words "death" and "dying" have little or no meaning to a child, even if he or she has experienced the death of a family member, a playmate, or a pet. This is true even

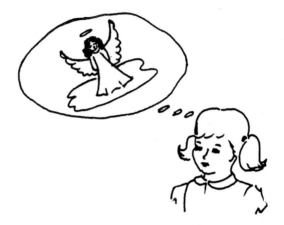

THINKING ABOUT DEATH

Figure 10-5.

if your child uses these words in conversation to describe fallen leaves, barren trees, or dead animals or insects around the house. Children of this young age have one prominent concern: fear of separation from their parents, family, friends, and home. Hospitalization, even if short, represents such a separation for a young child. Since he has little understanding of time, a few hours or a few days may seem like forever. For this reason, hospital policies generally make provision for extended or continuous parental visitation during both routine and serious hospital stays. This is not intended to encourage you to spend every moment of your child's various hospitalizations with him. If your child protests violently upon your leaving it may be because he thinks you are going forever. If you receive a bland greeting upon your return, your child may be displaying some anger over your absence. Both reactions are usually short-lived, but it is helpful to have your child talk about his feelings if he is mature enough to do so.

Understanding Death: 5-8 Years

Between the ages of five and eight years, there are two factors which make your child's understanding of death confused. The first of these is "reversibility," and the second is "magical thinking."

To a child of this age, *"reversibility"* means that you can be "dead" at one moment in time and alive at another time. For example, after having an elaborate burial in the backyard for a pet or other animal, the child may expect that same animal to be alive later. The child may worry about what the animal will eat and play with after it is dead and, thus, bury a bone or ball as well. Children's play often reflects their misperceptions of death. They play at being killed in "cops and robbers," falling down "dead" and then jumping up and continuing play. For them, being "dead" does not mean being out of the game permanently or, for that matter, for more than a few moments.

"*Magical thinking*" means that the child believes that thinking something is the same as doing it. For example, he might think, "I wish my sister was dead, because then I could have my own room." If this wish is followed within weeks or months by the actual death of the sibling, he may think he is directly responsible. This can produce overwhelming feelings of guilt and anxiety. The child might try to undo what he thinks he has done by saying, "I wished my sister would die so I could have my own room; but now, I wish God would give her back, because I'd rather have my sister again." Note both the sense of reversibility and the wishing in that statement.

However, some children feel too guilty about their fantasies to share them. If your child has never mentioned such thoughts, it might be helpful to introduce the subject yourself: "Son, some children might think it was their fault that their sister died. I wonder if sometimes you've had that feeling." Even if the child says no, it is appropriate to say something like: "I just wanted to make sure; because even though you and your sister had fights sometimes, her dying had nothing to do with you. I'm sure that she really liked the time you shared your special truck with her." You should be realistic about the occurrence of sibling rivalry and the feelings it arouses. Your child knows that these angry or jealous moments occurred and needs to be aware that you accept them. He should also be reassured by the fact that you remember and value the good parts of their interaction even more.

If your child needs more of your reassurance, he will bring up the subject again himself after he knows it is a "safe" topic. However, once may be enough for some children; and you should be sensitive to your individual child's needs to talk or not talk about any feelings of responsibility or remorse that he might have.

Similarly, for the sick child, "magical thinking" means that he feels that he has some control over his destiny and that events are directly related to his thoughts and actions. Thus, when faced with multiple painful or unpleasant procedures, he may believe that something he has thought or done has led to this "punishment."

Children at this age can be very difficult for parents to understand and manage. On the one hand, they talk about many things. On the other hand, they may not understand well enough to make even repeated explanations sufficient for their needs. Over and over again parents find themselves covering the same material, only to have their children ask the same questions in the same or slightly different form. Perhaps your exasperation can be lessened by understanding that the subject with which your child is being asked to deal is, in fact, beyond his comprehension. Keep your explanations short and simple and use such words as "dying," "death," and "dead" rather than "gone to sleep" or "gone on a trip." As you can imagine, if death is equated with sleep, children become afraid of monsters in the night or even of going into their bedrooms at all. Similarly, if death is equated with travel, trips become dreaded and are avoided if at all possible.

It is important to recognize that children do not have adult concepts of anxiety or sorrow about death. Instead, they are curious or matter-of-fact, and they oftentimes seem heartless. However, remember that sorrow is a response learned by experience and from watching and imitating adults. If a child seems to blurt out inappropriate comments or questions, or wants to play in the middle of serious discussions or times of crisis, it may not indicate a lack of caring but rather a lack of understanding. On the other hand, if his parents are sorrowful, the child may seek extra attention and cuddling for reassurance that everything will be all right. Alternatively, the child may try to comfort grieving adults — much as his parents comfort him when he is hurt.

Understanding Death: 9 Years and Older

By the age of about nine, most children begin to understand that death is an irreversible process, and their sense of time is mature enough to know that "forever" has some real meaning. The ability to rationalize and better understand what death means increases as they experience it through the loss of family members and friends.

There has been a tendency in American culture to shield children from death and not allow open discussion. Adults often mourn in private away from the young. Talking about the loss of someone close can bring people to the point of crying, even many years after the death. Thus, avoiding such discussion has become a general rule. Occasionally, parents become angry and upset when children talk about a dead brother or sister with little or no emotion. It is important to understand that the living child may have been quite young when his or her sibling died and remembrances may be vague. In addition, each person remembers differently; and it is important to allow children to have their own unique memories.

Lastly, "magical thinking" concerns about self-guilt persist in all of us, even through adulthood. Siblings may never share these feelings, or may share them only when they themselves are adults and have children of their own.

Talking with a Dying Child

For the dying child who is old enough to have even a rudimentary understanding of death, free and open discussion of concerns can be valuable. Perhaps the question which frightens people most, whether it comes from a child or an adult, is: "Am I going to die?" To be better able to answer that question in the future, stop and ask yourself what frightens you most about dying and death. In general, people answer that question in one of only a few different ways. The most common responses are fear of bodily hurt, loss of personal dignity, separation from loved ones, or nonfulfillment of some task or desired goal.

Children's concerns are similar to those of adults. When a child asks, "Am I going to die?", you might be tempted to give a yes or no answer. Yet such an answer does not give you an opportunity to know the child's understanding of death or his most pressing concerns. An alternative response could be: "I see that you have been thinking about dying. Tell me what is worrying you." This often produces answers which get at the very heart of the child's concerns or fears. For example, he might answer in one of these ways: "There will be nobody to take care of my puppy"; "I'm being stuck with needles all the time. Is it because I'm bad?"; or "I don't want Mommy or Daddy to leave me." When children are asked to share their thoughts directly, the answers that parents can give become more meaningful, because they relate to important issues for the child and give specific reassurance. Thus, the parents and child develop a sense of mutual understanding and communication that allows expression of both fear and love.

The important point to remember is that children differ in their understanding of dying and death. This understanding is directly related to their developmental level. As mentioned, the way you elect to go about discussing death depends upon your own background, experiences, and personal religious beliefs. The other children in your family also need to share this experience with you, because they are affected by it whether or not you discuss it openly with them. They will deal with the loss of a brother or sister more effectively if you help than if they are left to understand and cope on their own.

Sources of Help

Few parents feel emotionally able to manage their own feelings about the death of a child and the questions and concerns of the other children in the family as well. Sometimes, other family members can be valuable in helping parents cope. It may be wise to ask your child's doctor, one of the other health care professionals who know you and your family well, or a minister to give you some advice or assistance in understanding your child's concerns. Some parents ask various professionals to sit with them while they talk with their children. Other parents perfer to do this alone. Some parents find that their well children at home begin to ask questions before a sibling has died. Others find that many issues are not raised until weeks, months, or years afterwards.

When Do I Discuss Death with a Child?

The most appropriate time to give answers is when your child is asking questions. The most difficult task is to hear those questions when they are being asked. By being prepared, you will be a better listener and better able to support your child when the matter arises.

CHAPTER 11

HOSPITALIZATION

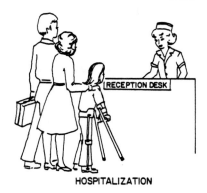

HOSPITALIZATION

Figure 11-1.

IT is important that parents understand what hospitalization means since children with spina bifida have a higher number of hospitalizations than the average child. Hospitalization includes a change to your child's surroundings, physical changes to his body, separation from family members, and interruption of his usual daily routine. This can be an especially stressing time for the entire family.

Hospital personnel are becoming increasingly more sensitive to the needs of children. Many hospitals have instituted a guided play program where children can act out some of their feelings through play. Yet hospitalization remains a difficult experience. An understanding of how your child may view the experience and how the family can be prepared for the event may help everyone deal with it better.

Planning for Hospitalization

Planning ahead for a hospital admission is particularly important for your child. Advance notice of this upcoming event can help him become accustomed to the idea. How far in advance you tell your child depends on his age. A three- or four-year-old can be told on the day of admission. Telling him sooner will not be helpful since he may not remember it. A four-to-six year-old can be gradually introduced to the idea one or two weeks before admission. Older children

99

can deal with several months of advance notice. Those between seven and 10 years of age may need to have the planned admission related to other events such as "after your birthday" or "before Christmas."

How detailed your preparation needs to be depends upon your child's age. Respond honestly and openly to any questions he may ask. This is the best way to provide the information that is important to him. Do not provide more information than he is really requesting, because his concerns may be very different from yours and much more basic. Listen to what is really being said and asked.

Many hospitals now have preadmission visits for children who will be admitted in the near future. These visits generally provide an opportunity for children and their parents to learn about the hospital and the likely experiences and people they will encounter. During such introductory sessions, you can ask such practical questions as what to take to the hospital and where parents can stay and eat. Children need to be at least four years old to benefit from this experience.

When an emergency hospital admission occurs, there is no opportunity to prepare. Both you and your child will probably be more nervous since there is no chance to plan. In addition, the illness itself may require a lot of your attention. You should realize that children in this circumstance have a special need to understand what is happening to them. A particular effort should be made to provide simple explanations, reassure fears and answer questions. Your ability to do this depends on the explanations you obtain and how you control your fears. You should seek out staff members who can tell you what is happening and support you in trying to help your child.

How the Rest of the Family Manages During Hospitalization

Your child will probably become the focus of attention for the whole family when he is hospitalized. Plans for other family actitivies often take second place to this child's needs. The first thing to consider is the affect of changes in household routine on the rest of the family as you attempt to satisfy the demands made on you both at the hospital and at home. The changes may be upsetting to the entire family, but especially so for younger brothers and sisters. They may find it hard to understand either the changes in routine or what is happening to their hospitalized brother or sister. This may result in generalized fears in the children at home.

Keeping meaningful contact with both your hospitalized child and those at home is important. Being away from home at important points like mealtimes can be minimized if you alternate eating in either setting. Both groups will understand if you present your schedule ahead of time. Planning alternate family activity times, rather than eliminating them entirely, can help keep life normal at home. Remember to *balance* the needs of both the hospitalized child and the children at home.

The children at home also need some type of contact with their hospitalized brother or sister. Parents can carry messages and mementos back and forth between them. This reassures them and encourages a sense of sharing and contact even during times of separation.

Common Responses to Hospitalization

Children often express their feelings about hospitalization in similar ways. Your child's age will play a major part in the way he acts before, during and after the hospital stay.

FEAR OF PARENTS LEAVING. Some children are particularly upset when their parents leave their side. This may be because they fail to understand that you will return again. They may feel your leaving the room is equivalent to your leaving their life forever. This is most common between the ages of two and four years. They do not understand explanations very well at this age. You should consider this age of "separation anxiety" to be an important period in which to spend time with a child who is hospitalized. Circumstances may make this difficult, but your presence has a special significance for a child at this age.

A LOSS OF PROGRESSIVE DEVELOPMENT. Regression is frequent during a prolonged hospitalization. It is common for children to *regress* when:

- They must remain in bed for long periods.
- They go long periods without seeing family faces.
- They are not stimulated by activities with other children in a playful environment.
- They have no opportunity to develop a substitute parent relationship with a member of the hospital staff.
- They cannot work out their feelings through meaningful play.

Children of any age can regress, but children from birth to two years of age are particularly susceptible. They may become quiet and lie silently in their crib for hours, especially when their cries are left unanswered. Often these children are mistakenly thought to be content. Toys and momentos from home to decorate your child's crib can help him feel secure with familiar items, as well as provide stimulation. Familiar items from home are reassuring.

Children in the hospital need to be kept active in normal daily activities or quiet play. Nurses try to encourage the children to continue doing things for themselves (dressing, feeding) which they did before coming to the hospital. When this is successful, it minimizes any loss of skills. This is particularly important for the child with spina bifida who already has faced the challenge of accomplishing tasks at the same time as his friends.

Parents should anticipate some regression in children once they return home. Understanding and gentle encouragement to continue with previously learned skills will help your child readjust in the shortest possible time.

FANTASY THINKING. Children have wonderful imaginations, and procedures or treatments can easily stimulate wild thoughts. Children between the ages of three and eight years are especially good at fantasies. They sometimes imagine that an object which punctures their skin will cause the inside of their body to leak out. If so, any needle puncture for blood tests or intravenous fluids will have special meaning. Preparation for procedures before they occur can help reduce such fears. Telling a child that a procedure is coming is often difficult for parents because it may result in very normal fussing and crying. You should remember that being surprised has a lasting effect on how much your child trusts you and others. A child should be told about a procedure a short time before it is performed. A matter-of-fact approach of explaining the procedure is best. Be honest about what will occur, how long it will last, and clearly state that it is necessary and cannot be avoided.

There is some debate as to whether parents should be in the room with the child when a procedure is performed. Some children are calmed by a parent's presence, while others cannot understand why the parent is not rescuing them from their plight. In addition, some parents are calm and understanding, while others are tense, nervous, and more upset than the child. If you fall in the latter category, your presence may make it more difficult for both your child and the staff. The judgement to stay or leave should be made jointly by you and the hospital staff. The staff does expect you to make it clear to your child that the decision to perform the procedure rests with them. This will enable you to be a comforting parent and not confuse your child about who decided that the procedure needed to be done.

FEAR OF DEATH. This is common for young children, but dying is usually not thought of in the same way as adults view it. Children may think of it as a temporary problem. It is probable that such thoughts occur to children who feel they are in danger.

Children with spina bifida are generally not in situations where their life is in danger for long time periods. However, you should be alert to any signals that your child is worried about his well-being. These worries are often based on misunderstandings about how their body works. For instance, a teenager facing back surgery may worry that his lungs will pop like a balloon if the surgeon slips with the knife. The fact that surgeons are careful people and that lungs are not like balloons could be reassuring information that he needs to hear.

A FEELING OF BEING BAD AND, THEREFORE, RESPONSIBLE FOR THE HOSPITALIZATION. This feeling is common in children between the ages of four and ten years. The child may feel that since his body caused the hospitalization, it must be his fault. People are punished for being bad, so he must have been very bad indeed. In addition, when he notes that his parents are upset about the hospitalization, he may assume he is also responsible for their anxiety. Parents need to be particularly reassuring on this issue.

Many of these fears may combine during a hospital stay. *Acting out* or creating a behavior disturbance is an expression of this anxiety. This is common for children five years of age and older. Some protest about what is happening is a healthy response; but if it is allowed to continue or becomes excessive, it can be the source of even greater anxiety in itself. This is the time when parents and others should restate the rules of conduct, or distract the younger child into meaningful play and engage the older child in discussion about their understanding of what is happening.

Rooming-in by Parents

Twenty-four hour visiting for parents is widespread now, but only a decade ago visiting on children's units was discouraged. Some hospitals now have accommodations where a parent can stay with a child at night. These accommodations vary but usually consist of a cot or day bed in the child's room.

How much time you spend with your child while he is in the hospital should depend upon such things as his age, needs, condition and other demands on your time. The admission literature from the hospital will generally tell you about the accomodations for parents, and you can make preliminary arrangements. These can be discussed with the nursing and medical staff at the time of admission.

If you plan to stay, it is wise to have some books or other materials that will help you pass the hours when your child is sleeping or otherwise occupied. You should limit this material, however, since space is often limited in hospitals.

If You Cannot Stay with Your Child

Many factors may prevent you from staying with your child in the hospital. If you cannot stay, careful planning will make it possible for you to be with him at the most important times. There are two periods when your child will probably find it particularly helpful for you to be present. The first is when difficult, frightening, or uncomfortable activities or treatments are scheduled. The second is during the day or night when important family events routinely occur at home. Mealtimes and bedtime often have a special significance to children. A discussion with your child's nurse may help you in deciding at which times it would be most beneficial for you to visit. Even though your child will be cared for in your absence, your contact and availability to him continue to be important, especially at key times. Together, you and the hospital staff form the best team in caring for him.

What to Expect from the Nursing Staff

Your child will be cared for by several nurses during his hospitalization. Because nurses work in shifts of about eight hours, at least three different nurses will work with your child in a twenty-four hour period. It appears best if the nurses caring for your child on one day continue with his care on subsequent days. This continuity of contact between your child and a nurse allows both to develop a knowledgeable and trusting relationship. This arrangement is not always possible but you should make a special request if it does not happen.

Nursing assignments in many hospitals, especially university centers, are organized so that one nurse is responsible for each child's overall plan of nursing care. She is called the primary nurse. Other nurses may take over in her absence, but they would follow her plan. This plan is developed for your child when he is admitted and will be updated as his needs change. The information you provide the primary nurse regarding your child's schedules, habits, abilities and individual differences will be helpful when the plan is developed. This primary nurse system is not present in all hospitals. It seems desirable, but competent nursing can be provided even in its absence.

On each hospital floor, there is a coordinator of nursing activities. That coordinator is referred to as the head nurse, the nurse clinician, or the charge nurse. She can help you by answering questions related to the overall activities of the unit. When a problem arises it is generally best to go first to your child's primary nurse. She will know if further help or advice is needed.

Although nurses caring for your child will have studied the problems of the child with spina bifida, they may not have had extensive exposure to children with this defect. Therefore, information regarding the specific care for your child's needs may be helpful to the nurse. She can work with you to devise the best overall plan of care for your child.

The Medical Staff

Just as your child will have contact with many nurses, several physicians will also be involved in his care while he is in the hospital. The type of physicians will depend upon the nature of the problem for which he is hospitalized and the type of hospital he enters.

Although multiple specialists may be in contact with your child, only one physician will be listed as his attending physician. Whether he is a surgeon, neurologist, pediatrician or some other specialist, he is the person responsible for your child's overall medical care while in the hospital. This attending physician will admit, administer to, and discharge your child under his personal supervision. Other specialists may provide consultation for various aspects of your chlid's medical care, but all major decisions are the responsibility of the attending physician. He should explain to you the need for any consultations.

In teaching hospitals, there will usually be an intern and resident pediatricians (house officers). They will also play a major role in caring for your child. This is especially true in a university medical center. These professionals are fully qualified and licensed physicians who are receiving specialty training. They will examine your child and follow his progress with the attending physician. They should be well-informed about your child's condition and can usually be reached more easily than the attending physician. They can talk to the many specialists and keep you informed about how others see your child's progress. It is important that they and the attending physician communicate with each other so that you receive advice upon which they agree.

If your child has surgery, there may also be a surgical resident involved in his care. He may be from urology, orthopedics, neurosurgery, or another specialty. He will work closely with your child's attending physician, who will be a surgeon in this case. The surgical resident is generally more available than the attending surgeon.

The different physicians and personnel caring for your child will try to keep you informed, but the times they visit your child may not coincide with your visits. Your child's pediatric house officer or nurse can help you contact the attending physician or other specialists, if they cannot provide an answer. Let them know your questions and concerns.

Coordination of Hospital Services

While your child is in the hospital, an effort will be made to schedule treatments, tests, and procedures at times which are convenient for your child. Because multiple services within the hospital must be utilized, schedules often need to be adjusted to coincide with the available resources. For example, not all surgery can be performed at 8:00 AM and not all physiotherapy carried out at 10:00 AM, although these times might be most convenient for some patients or families.

Often multiple, specialized services are needed for the hospitalized child with spina bifida. The coordination of these services is time-consuming. Answers to parents' questions sometimes need to wait until information from tests and procedures has been received and several professionals have had an opportunity to communicate. This process occasionally means that parents need to wait for decisions, and often that dates for events such as surgery and discharge are arranged close to the time they take place.

Getting Ready to Go Home

There is an increasing trend to send children home at the earliest possible moment. The cost of hospitalization today is one of the reasons, but also the health professions have rediscovered that home is where children usually do best. For this reason, you may find your child still needs some form of treatment at home. Generally, this is the kind of care that the staff feels a parent can provide; but sometimes the periodic help of a public health nurse will also be needed. If the care at home is going to be more complicated, assistance in your home may be available through your local Public Health or Visiting Nurse Agency or Home Care Association. Before your child is discharged, the staff will help you make these plans and teach you how to provide the needed care. You should discuss with the staff your child's needs after discharge well before the final day. This will give you adequate time to make plans and prepare for the return home. Your child's nurse, working with the unit social worker, can assist you most in making these plans.

Working with the Staff During Times of Hospitalization

The principles, which appear in the chapter on working with the specialty team, also apply to working with personnel during hospitalization. In most health care institutions the same personnel work in both inpatient and outpatient settings. Their roles may differ slightly in each area. In order for you to know what to expect from any individual, you must understand the roles of the different specialists. The following is a list of the various professionals you may encounter either in the hospital or on outpatient visits. How many different professionals you may encounter will depend on your child's difficulties, the size of your hospital, whether it is associated with a medical center and the extent of any spina bifida team.

Audiologist
Dietitian/Nutritionist
Enterostomal Therapist
Family Counselor
Inhalation Therapist
Nurses
    Practical Nurse
    Registered Nurse
    Head Nurse

Nurse Clinical Specialist
Nurse Practitioner
Public Health or Visiting Nurse
Primary Nurse
Nurse's Aide
Occupational Therapist
Orthotist
Physical Therapist
Physicians
    Intern   Urologist
    Resident   Gastroenterologist
    Pediatrician   Geneticist
    Orthopedist   Infectious Disease
    Neurologist   Family Practitioner
    Neurosurgeon   General Practitioner
Opthalmologist
Prosthetist
Psychologist
School Teacher
Secretary
Social Worker
Speech Therapist or Pathologist
Students

Section II

Understanding How Your Child's Body Functions

CHAPTER 12

THE OPEN SPINE

A CLOSER LOOK AT THE OPEN SPINE

SPINA BIFIDA is readily apparent at birth. Although the open spine is easily seen and diagnosed, evaluating the seriousness in an individual child is more difficult. Physicians and others who are experienced in dealing with children having this defect usually view it more optimistically than do others who deal with it less frequently.

How the Back Appears at Birth

The opening in the spine may be at any spot, but it is most often in the lower back.

It may have a smooth covering of skin, or there may be no skin over the deeper tissues. If skin covers the opening it may be normal or thin and delicate. When skin does not cover the opening, the delicate coverings of the spinal cord are usually visible. Accompanying these coverings is often a pinkish tissue which is incorrectly developed spinal cord.

The coverings over the open spine may be bulging and form a lump on the back or they may be fairly flat. The fluid which surrounds the spinal cord and brain is held in by these coverings, and this accounts for the swelling. If this fluid leaks out, the membranes do not bulge.

The opening in the spine may be very small or quite extensive. Usually the defect is two to four inches in length. Rarely is the entire spine open. Although the bulging skin or delicate spinal cord coverings may be large, the most important point in determining the extent of the defect relates to how many of the underlying bones of the spine (vertebra) are incorrectly formed.

The Different Types of Spina Bifida

Meningocoele
Myelomeningocoele (Meningomyelocoele)
Spina bifida occulta

It will help you to understand the common types of spina bifida if you know what the parts of each word mean.

111

Meningo means meninges or the delicate coverings which surround the spinal cord and brain (nervous system).

Myelo means spinal cord or the nerve tissue which is protected by the bones of the spine.

Coel means sac. In this instance it is the cavity which is filled with the fluid that surrounds the spinal cord and brain (spinal fluid or cerebrospinal fluid).

Occulta means hidden or not readily apparent.

A *meningocoele* is thus a type of spina bifida where there is a sac which contains only the meninges. There is no spinal cord in the sac and, therefore, the baby is not likely to have the same disabilities as in myelomeningocele.

A *myelomeningocoele* may have a large sac or a flat open area. The defect contains spinal cord in addition to the meninges. Most of the children with spina bifida have this type and consequently have some nerve tissue which is not working properly. This entire book deals primarily with children who have this specific type of spina bifida.

Spina bifida occulta is a hidden defect and, although present at birth, is not usually seen. There is simply a minor defect in the bones of the spine. When this type of defect is present, there may be a birthmark or a patch of hair over the area of the spine where the defect occurs. A hidden spina bifida is more common; and most of the children who have it are entirely without disability. This is because the spinal cord is not usually involved.

How Can the Type of Spina Bifida be Determined?

When a spina bifida is seen at birth, it is most often a myelomeningocoele. Usually this defect is the type which does not have skin covering it. The incorrectly formed spinal cord and related nerve tissue can usually be seen lying on the surface of the open spine.

When the spina bifida is covered with skin, it may be difficult to decide if the spinal cord is involved or not. If there is paralysis of any muscles in the legs, then the nerve tissue is definitely involved. When no paralysis is seen, there is a good chance that the infant has a *meningocoele*. However, this diagnosis can only be made when the surgeon who repairs the defect looks to see if there is nervous tissue within the sac.

How Does the Spina Bifida Affect Your Child's Function?

Normally, the spinal cord gives off a series of nerves that provide pathways for receiving in and sending out messages from the brain. The brain usually gets messages from all the various parts of the body and then sends out messages telling the body parts what they should do. In spina bifida these messages are not being transmitted back and forth in the proper way. The abnormal nervous tissue in the spina

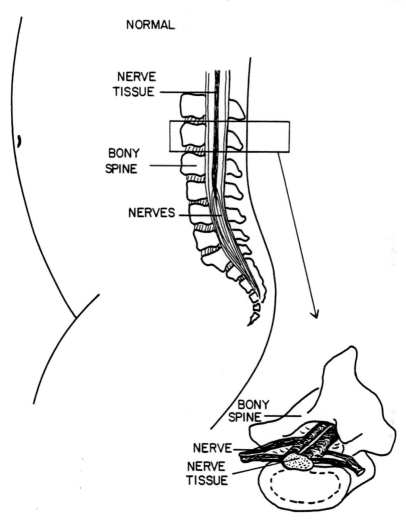

NORMAL

NERVE
TISSUE

BONY
SPINE

NERVES

BONY
SPINE

NERVE

NERVE
TISSUE

Figure 12-1.

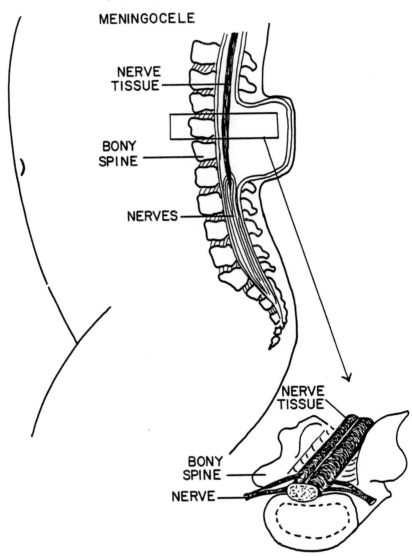

MENINGOCELE

NERVE
TISSUE

BONY
SPINE

NERVES

NERVE
TISSUE

BONY
SPINE

NERVE

Figure 12-2.

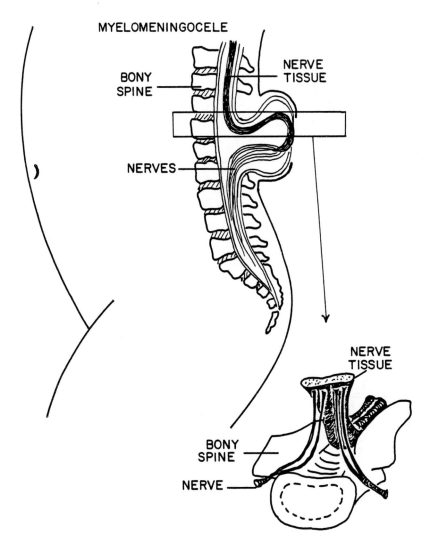

Figure 12-3.

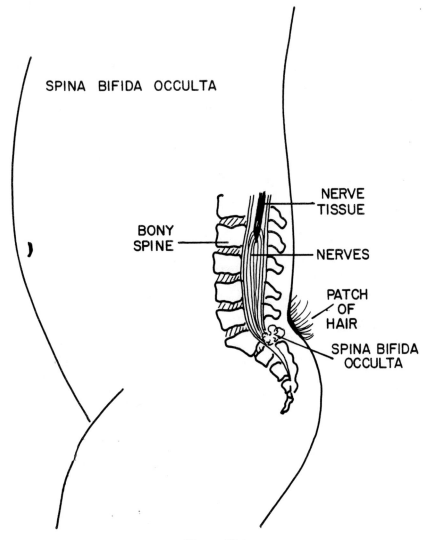

Figure 12-4.

bifida itself acts as a barrier in the transmission of these messages.

Messages *sent out* usually go to the muscles. This is the way we control movements and keep from urinating or having a bowel movement, except when we so desire. These messages are organized so that nerves from different areas of the spinal cord control different groups of muscles. Fortunately, there is stimulation of the most important muscles by nerves from several areas of the spinal cord. This means that if one nerve does not work, the child may still retain some control over that muscle if another nerve to that muscle is functioning.

The messages that are *received* by nerve tissue are the various *feelings* such as pain, temperature, touch, etc. These messages are also organized by areas, but there is not much overlap in the areas from which these feelings arise. When a nerve does not work, usually all the feeling is lost in the area from which it brings messages.

Your child's ability to function will be affected by his degree of paralysis. Paralysis results when the messages from the brain do not reach the body to tell it what it should do. When the messages are blocked the muscles do not move when the brain wants them to. Sometimes paralysis is associated with a lack of feeling also. That is, the brain does not receive the messages about what is happening to the body. In spina bifida the paralysis is often associated with loss of feeling. The loss of both movement and feeling usually involves only the lower half of the body. This may include the stomach muscles and muscles along the spine or in the hips, legs and feet. The muscles that allow voluntary control of the urine and stool are usually paralyzed too.

What Determines How Much Paralysis Is Present?

The area of the spine where the open spine begins is the most important determinant of how much paralysis occurs. Most open spines occur in the lower back (lumbar area), but some occur below this in the area of the tailbone (sacral area). Occasionally they occur higher up on the back or even the neck (thoracic or cervical). How often spina bifida occurs in each area of the spine is shown in the accompanying figure. The parts of the body below the open spine are subject to either partial or complete paralysis. Paralysis does not occur above the level of the open spine. Spina bifida which occurs on the high back or neck is sometimes of the meningocoele type and does not affect the nerve tissue under it.

Most defects are two to four inches (5 to 10 centimeters) in length. They usually involve three or four vertebral bones, but can be smaller or larger. The larger the defect, the more spinal cord and nerve tissue that will likely be affected. The most common defects usually occur in the lumbar area. They may span several inches and extend into the thoracic or sacral area.

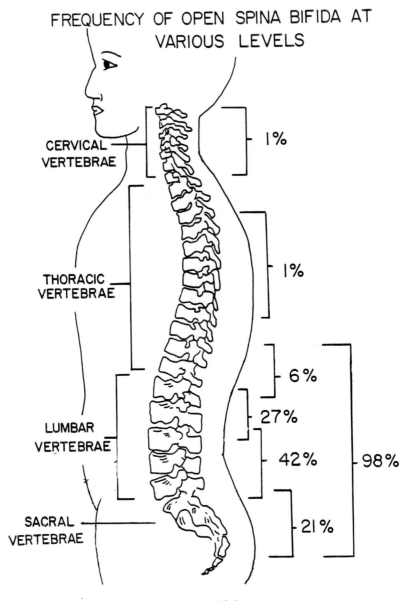

FREQUENCY OF OPEN SPINA BIFIDA AT VARIOUS LEVELS

CERVICAL VERTEBRAE — 1%

THORACIC VERTEBRAE — 1%

LUMBAR VERTEBRAE — 6%, 27%, 42%, 98%

SACRAL VERTEBRAE — 21%

Figure 12-5.

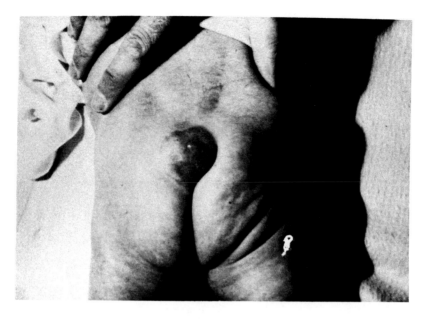

Skin-covered Spina Bifida.

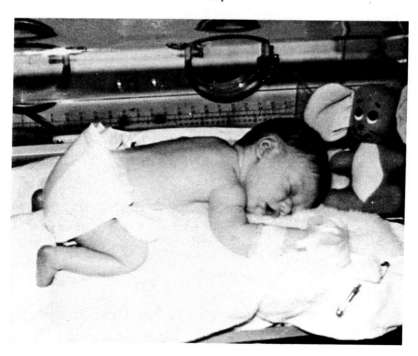

The Individual Patterns of Nerve Tissue Affected

Although children with spina bifida appear similar, there are individual differences in the patterns of nerve tissue involvement. This accounts for the varying degrees of paralysis in children with spina bifida. Even those who have spinal defects at similar levels and of the same size may be very different in how they function. A careful neurological examination is needed to determine your child's individual pattern.

One confusing factor is that some muscles may be paralyzed in a tense or tight (spastic) manner, and others paralyzed in a limp or relaxed (flaccid) manner. When the paralyzed muscles are spastic, movements may appear when the leg or toes are touched or stimulated. When these movements occur, the child is usually not aware of them and is unable to control them. If the stimulation is painful, he will not feel it. These spastic or tight muscles can cause a steady pull on bones and lead to orthopedic problems. By contrast the flaccid muscles do not move or pull. When normal or spastic muscles affect the same bone or joint as flaccid ones, the unbalanced forces will lead to orthopedic problems. Any combination of these neurological difficulties may be present in a child with spina bifida, and only careful evaluation of the individual child can determine his particular pattern.

It is important to remember that spina bifida is a problem which occurs when the baby is being formed. Since many types of nerve tissue are developing in the fetus at one time, many areas of nervous tissue may be affected at the same time in different ways. Some of these areas may not be normal, but they still may be able to function, often quite well. In contrast to spina bifida which occurs when the nervous system does not develop correctly, a great deal of the medical information on spinal cord problems has been gained by studying other conditions such as spinal cord trauma. This can lead to a confusion, particularly when the child's progress is better than people expect.

The Danger of Infection

The open spine presents an easy way for germs to enter the spinal fluid which bathes the spinal cord and brain. Once germs are in this fluid, they can grow and spread very quickly. If there is a protective covering of the skin over the open spine, it is more difficult for the germs to enter. When the spinal fluid is leaking through the sac from the open spine, the germs can travel up this pathway and enter the body. When the spinal fluid is leaking, the risk of infection is very high.

When the infection is in the spinal fluid it can spread around the spinal cord, brain and meninges. This is termed *meningitis*. If this infection spreads to the spaces inside the brain called ventricles, it is termed *ventriculitis*. Either of these infections is very serious. If untreated these infections are usually fatal. Both types of infection require early and vigorous treatment if the child is to be given the best opportunity for the future.

The Value of Repairing the Back

The major reason for repairing the back is to decrease the chances of infection. The repair will also make the infant easier to handle. No matter how darling a child is, an obvious birth defect detracts from the way people interact with him. Both you and they will be concerned about holding and touching him. Before the operation the infant may be unable to lie on his back. Since all infants need love, which includes holding and cuddling, it is helpful to have the baby in the most "holdable" condition. When you can easily handle your infant, your view of him should improve. Other people will also view him more favorably.

Although the operation to repair the baby's back will do many positive things, it will not cure the infant. The operation will not improve how well the spinal cord and nerve tissue function. Usually there is no further loss of function. The benefits of this surgery are important to your child's future.

What Will Happen If the Back Is Not Repaired?

Normally after birth the skin begins to grow over the open spine, and after a few weeks or months there will be a covering over the sac. This skin is often a thin delicate covering and it can easily tear and leak spinal fluid. Sometimes the skin covering the sac is thicker and then there is less danger of leakage.

Studies show that children with a *serious* type of spina bifida, who do not have back surgery, are likely to die in the first year of life. Most of these children die from infections.

If your child has a serious form of spina bifida and a decision is made not to repair the back, he will most likely die. If the spina bifida is a less serious type, then whether or not the back is repaired he will probably survive. Even knowing this, some parents who love their child with spina bifida support the decision not to have surgery. A decision not to repair the back is usually confined to children with the severe form of spina bifida, where those involved feel that having the child live with a severe debilitating spina bifida is not fair to either the child or the family. Many people face this same crisis when older loved ones have serious illnesses from which they can never fully recover or cannot be saved. When the decision is reached not to surgically correct the open spine, some families prefer to take their child home. At home they can share that one thing that the child and the family need most, love.

The decisions most families reach are heavily influenced by the attitudes of the physician and others caring for their infant. It is important that you have confidence in those individuals and their ability to help you reach the right decision. If you lack confidence, you have every right to seek another opinion. Occasionally families do this even if they completely trust the judgment of those caring for the baby. This is an important decision and one which will affect the lives of you, your child, your family, and others around you for many years. Most children who have spina bifida are not so seriously impaired, and the decision to surgically repair the back is easier to reach.

What Is the Best Time to Repair the Back?

When the operation on the back should be done is not an easy question to answer. For many years doctors felt that immediate repair of the back would prevent further nerve tissue damage and infants underwent operations within a few hours of birth. This does not appear to be true, and doctors now feel that nearly all of the damage is already present at birth.

Before the operation on the open spine occurs, a discussion with the family and an evaluation of the infant needs to take place. In addition, technical decisions about the operation must be made. A discussion with the family is essential so they will understand what the defect means and can begin to cope with the problems it presents. Both parents should be involved whenever possible. The family, of course, must also give permission for the operation.

The evaluation of the infant with spina bifida has already been described (see Evaluating the Baby and Making Decisions). If certain problems are evident at birth, they may influence the recommendations of those caring for your child. Hydrocephalus, kidney damage, a total paralysis below the waist, a marked curve or bend in the spine and other birth defects not usually associated with spina bifida are examples of such complicating problems.

The technical decisions relate to the size of the open back and how best to repair it. Occasionally a delay of several weeks allows the skin to grow around the opening and makes repair easier. This must be weighed against the possibility of infection, the problems of handling the infant, and the family's view of the child. Leakage of fluid from the back would be an important reason for doing the repair as soon as possible. Another technical problem arises if the infant has hydrocephalus (too much fluid under pressure within the head). When this is present, some doctors feel it should be corrected before the back is repaired. Usually surgical repair of the back is accomplished in the first few days of life.

The Risks of the Operation

Tests to determine how well nerve tissue functions in a newborn are difficult, and techniques are not presently available to determine small differences in individual muscles or nerves. However, with present techniques, repair of the open spine usually does not cause more damage to the nervous system than was present at birth.

The infant must be anesthetized for this operation, and there is always a small risk that complications will be associated with anesthesia. In addition, there is a small risk of infection ocurring at the operative site. Generally, the risks of complication are quite small.

How the Back Looks After Repair

Following closure of the defect and healing of the surgical incision, there will be a scar. The shape and size of your child's scar will depend upon what is required by the surgeon to close the open spine. Often the skin around the scar is red, and this may spread out from the scar for several inches. This is like a birthmark and has no significance. Sometimes there will also be hair growing from the skin around the scar. This hair is usually long, dark and distinctly different from other hair on the back. Once the open spine is repaired, it cannot occur again in that child.

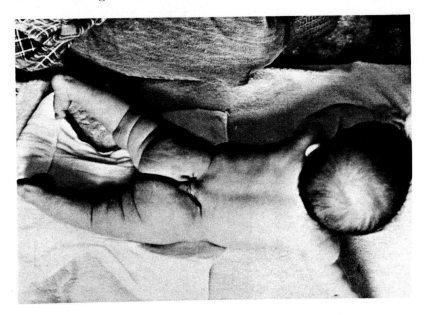

Figure 12-6. Healed scar after spina bifida repair.

How the Surgery Is Performed

The operation consists of putting the infant to sleep, carefully removing the lump, and then bringing the skin together over the defect. The surgeon cuts around the edges of the sac and removes both the sac and its covering of thin skin. The sac is next carefully removed with every effort given to saving as much of the spinal cord and nerve tissue within the sac as possible. After removal of the sac, the deep tissues are carefully put together so that the fluid around the nerve tissue does not leak under the skin or through the wound. The skin is then loosened around the edges and the edges of the skin pulled together and joined. If the defect is large, sometimes a flap of skin will be moved over it. The surgeon then places a skin graft over the neighboring area from which the skin flap was taken.

With very large defects, it is sometimes medically best to wait until the skin around the defect grows thicker before closing the opening. At times defects are so large that waiting for more skin growth is the only solution.

The Unrepaired Back

There are many reasons why an infant with spina bifida might come home with an unrepaired back defect. Families with an infant in this condition are called upon to develop a practical means of managing the defect on the back as well as a comfortable way of holding their newborn.

A means of protecting your baby's back from bumps and jars is what is needed. Whatever protection is used must be easy to change and keep clean, not too cumbersome, and allow the child to be held easily without affecting the defect.

Dressing the Back

Several answers to this problem have been devised. One of the simplest and most successful is a ring made of clean cotton wadding and wrapped in gauze. This ring encircles the defect and protects it. The ring can help hold small dressing pads which are placed directly over the defect. In some cases these dressings may need to be kept moistened with a sterile water solution. This will prevent the dressing sticking to the skin and keep the skin soft rather than allowing it to dry. The ring and dressings can be kept in place by devices called Montgomery straps. An adhesive strip is attached on either side of the baby's back below the defect. Strings attached to the adhesive then come up and tie over the ring and dressings to secure them snugly in place. The dressing will need to be changed two to three times a day.

With Mom and Dad using clean hands, the ring can be changed every one to two days or depending on how soiled it gets. Montgomery straps can stay on for three to four days at a time, if the adhesive is not too irritating to the skin. You will need to modify your child's clothing sizes to accommodate the increased bulk from the dressings.

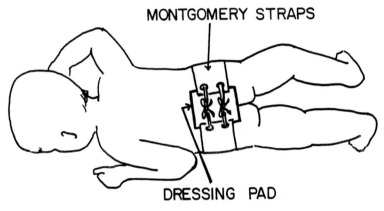

Figure 12-7.

Positioning

The baby can be positioned lying on either side or on his abdomen. He can be held upright in your arms or sit in your lap. Lying flat on his back for the time being will not be possible.

It will be necessary to make sure that stool and urine do not come in contact with the defect on the back. Keeping your baby's back a little lower than his head will help the urine and stool drain in the right direction. A small plastic sheet attached below the open spine can also be used to prevent any stool from accidentally getting on the dressing.

What Should You Watch for?

When you change the protective dressings, be alert for signs which need to be reported to your doctor.

Leakage of spinal fluid

Red streaks, swelling or unusual warmth around the defect

A change in the shape or size of the defect

After the Back Is Repaired

After the defect has been repaired and the scar is healed, the baby can be placed on his back for brief periods. The time can be gradually increased as the skin heals, but he should probably sleep on his abdomen for the first several weeks after surgery.

CHAPTER 13

THE HEAD

THE bones of the skull protect the brain. At birth these bones are not joined together, but as a child grows they become firmly attached to each other. Usually by two years of age they are difficult to separate.

The brain is surrounded by a clear fluid that looks like water. This fluid is called spinal fluid and it also fills the spaces within the brain. The spaces within the brain are usually small and are called ventricles. There are five of them and the fluid in each can move to any other. This fluid is made inside the ventricles, and then flows through other ventricles and passageways and finally circulates over the brain and spinal cord. It is this same fluid that fills the sac on the back when there is a spina bifida. This fluid eventually passes into the bloodstream. About a pint (500 cc) of fluid is produced and reabsorbed by the bloodstream each day.

What Changes Are Associated with Spina Bifida?

Most infants with spina bifida have hydrocephalus. In some children, however, careful observation may be the only treatment required.

Children with spina bifida often have an unusual structural change of the brain which is called the Arnold-Chiari malformation. This happens when the brain is developing. It can be associated with several problems. In this malformation a part of the lower end of the brain is partially lying inside the neck vertebrae. This does not normally happen. Because of this there may be a blockage to the spinal fluid as it tries to flow out of the brain so it can be reabsorbed by the bloodstream. When this malformation is present blockage can also occur at other places, such as the aqueduct, within the brain. The Arnold-Chiari malformation is commonly associated with spina bifida. Children who have meningocoeles or spina bifida very low on the back, on the neck, or high on the trunk may not have it. These children may not have hydrocephalus either.

What Is Hydrocephalus?

This term means that the spaces inside the brain (ventricles) are larger than usual. These spaces are always filled with spinal fluid, so the term hydrocephalus means the brain has too much spinal fluid

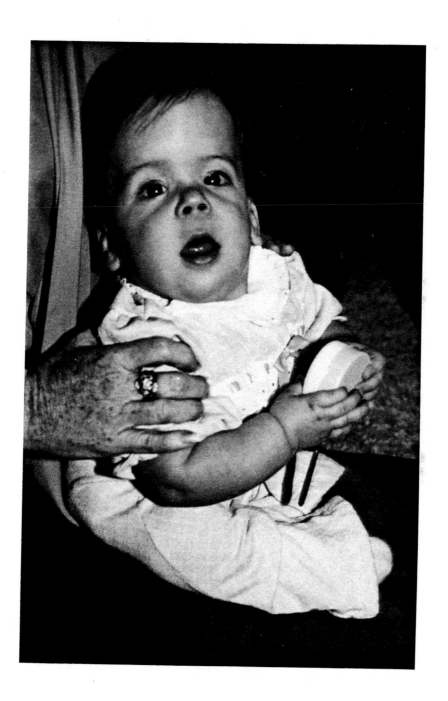

within its ventricles.

Whenever there is obstruction to the flow of spinal fluid or its return to the bloodstream, hydrocephalus will result. This fluid is constantly being formed inside the ventricles and must continuously flow out of the brain and be reabsorbed. If this flow and reabsorption does not occur, then the fluid will accumulate and enlarge the spaces within the brain.

The Two Types of Hydrocephalus

Blockage to the flow of spinal fluid can occur either inside or outside the brain. This leads to two basic kinds of hydrocephalus: (A) communicating and (B) noncommunicating. If the spinal fluid is blocked from getting to the outside of the brain it is noncommunicating hydrocephalus. The spaces inside the brain (ventricles) do not communicate with the spaces outside. If the fluid reaches the outside of the brain but cannot be reabsorbed into the bloodstream, then it is called communicating hydrocephalus.

THE NORMAL FLUID SPACES
WITHIN THE BRAIN

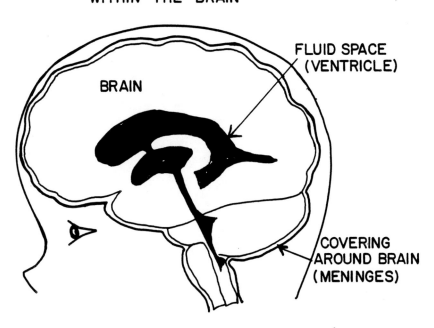

Figure 13-1.

THE FLUID SPACES IN THE BRAIN WITH
HYDROCEPHALUS AND THE USUAL AREAS
OF BLOCKAGE.

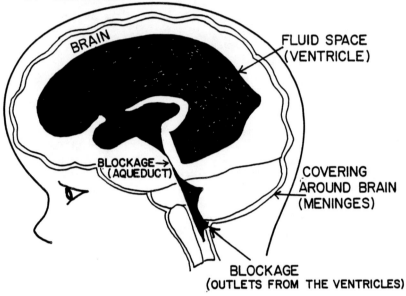

Figure 13-2.

Causes of Noncommunicating Hydrocephalus

Blockage of spinal fluid so that it cannot leave the ventricles of the brain can occur at several places. Each of the ventricles normally communicates with the others by a narrow passage or opening. The most common place for blockage to occur is a narrow passageway called the aqueduct. Another common area of blockage is where the fluid leaves the ventricles to pass into the spaces around the brain. These openings normally form as the brain is developing. They may fail to develop or develop incompletely in the child with the Arnold-Chiari malformation.

Causes of Communicating Hydrocephalus

Spinal fluid normally leaves the ventricles at the bottom end of the brain. The fluid then travels up over the brain and is reabsorbed into the bloodstream at the top. Obstruction to this reabsorption can occur in the Arnold-Chiari malformation. This type of obstruction may also follow spinal fluid infections or bleedings.

How to Tell If Hydrocephalus Is Present

Most infants with spina bifida have hydrocephalus. It may be difficult to tell if there is hydrocephalus until the head size (the head circumference is measured the same as for a hat) enlarges, or until special tests such as a CAT, EMI or other special x-ray tests are done. Carefully following the head size is one of the easiest and most reliable ways of detecting progressive hydrocephalus. Normally head growth follows a schedule; but when the growth is faster than expected for the child's age, there is serious concern about the degree of hydrocephalus present. Repeated special x-ray studies can provide similar information; but infants often must be sedated, and the difficulty and expense of these studies is much greater than simply measuring the head.

Getting the correct head measurement from a squirming child is sometimes difficult. Since important decisions may rest on this measurement, it should be done accurately by your family doctor, public health nurse or other specialists.

Hydrocephalus Differs with Age

Skull bones can move apart easily in infants up until one year of age. When pressure inside the ventricles becomes too much, the bones are forced to spread apart, thereby relieving the pressure on the brain. This spreading of the bones is what leads to a gradual enlargement of the head. This is nature's way of reducing pressure. In the child less than one year old, this reduction in pressure makes hydrocephalus a less urgent concern. In the older children, whose bones do not separate easily, small changes in pressure can quickly lead to serious problems.

How Can You Tell If the Pressure Is Too High?

There are several things that you may notice if hydrocephalus is present. They result from too much fluid and, therefore, pressure in the ventricles. The "soft spot" on top of the head may bulge and feel firm. The head size may increase. The skin over the skull may appear shiny and the veins appear very distinct. The eyes may turn downward so that the white shows above the colored iris. If the child is old enough to talk, he may complain of headache. Younger children who presumably have a headache may be irritable, awaken from sleep, or simply hold their head and shake it. Vomiting may occur, especially in the morning. After vomiting the child may even be able to eat breakfast. Vomiting may also occur after eating. This type of vomiting is usually sudden and the child does not feel nauseated or sick in the stomach before vomiting.

As the pressure increases further sleepiness occurs. Initially the child may be hard to arouse and quickly doze off again. Later he cannot even be aroused.

The three main symptoms of hydrocephalus which require that you take action very soon are:

Sleepiness (unable to awaken)
Vomiting (usually repeatedly)
Irritability

If you notice other features of hydrocephalus, you should call them to your doctor's attention; but they do not require such urgent action.

Occasionally hydrocephalus is very mild and may progress so slowly that there will not be any of these changes apparent in your child. This can occur at most ages but is especially true in small children. The brain is able to adapt to small changes which occur over a long period of time. When this occurs, head measurements, examination of the eyes, or laboratory tests may help your physician to recognize what is occurring.

The health team may need more information about your child's brain at some point in time, but a great deal of information can be gained by looking at the brain in various indirect ways. The following tests are used to gain information about the brain. Detailed information about the brain is especially important if surgery is planned or being considered.

SKULL X-RAYS. These look at the bones which surround the brain. If the bones are separated, this is a sign of increased pressure inside the head. Sometimes the bones are thin and infants with spina bifida often have skull bones which are very distinctive on x-rays. Taking these x-rays requires careful positioning of the head. There is no particular discomfort.

CAT SCAN. (Computerized axial tomography, EMI) — This is a special study that gives a picture of how the inside of the brain appears. It can show the size of the ventricles. A computer averages the same point in space on many x-ray beams directed through the head and then reconstructs an image. The child must lie very still for several minutes, and small children must sometimes be sedated or occasionally anesthetized. Some newer machines are much faster and the child may not even need sedation. The test is not painful.

SPINAL TAP (LP, LUMBAR PUNCTURE). This test looks directly at the spinal fluid. It can reveal information about the pressure inside the head and detect infection in this fluid. The procedure is uncomfortable, because the child must stay in a certain position while the fluid is removed. In addition, there is a needle stick in the back.

PNEUMOENCEPHALOGRAM (PEG). This study consists of doing a spinal tap and injecting air. The air rises and enters the ventricles showing the spaces in and around the brain very well. The air is eventually absorbed and does not leave any after-effects. The children are anesthetized for this procedure.

VENTRICULOGRAM. In this test, a needle is placed through the brain and air is injected directly into the ventricles. This avoids any change in spinal fluid pressure which can result if the air is introduced through a spinal tap. If the ventricles do not connect (noncommunicating hydrocephalus) with the spaces outside the brain, then air must be placed directly into them if they are to be visualized. The child is anesthetized for this procedure.

CEREBRAL ARTERIOGRAM. This is a special x-ray study of the blood vessels to the brain. It is seldom necessary in children with spina bifida. It consists of injecting a special material into the blood vessels to the head and, thus, outlining exactly where those blood vessels lie. In conditions such as hydrocephalus, they do not lie in a normal position. Children are anesthetized for this procedure.

BRAIN SCAN. This test consists of injecting a harmless radioactive material into the bloodstream. If blood vessels in the brain are abnormal, they will permit this material to enter the brain, but normal blood vessels do not. After injecting the material, a special type of x-ray detects its distribution. The injection is the most uncomfortable part of the procedure.

RISA SCAN. This is a special test where a spinal tap is done and a harmless radioactive substance injected. Spinal fluid circulates around the brain and, by using special x-ray equipment, the movement of the radioactive material can be followed. The only discomfort is the spinal tap required to introduce the radioactive substance.

ELECTROENCEPHALOGRAM (EEG). This test measures the electrical activity that the brain produces. Small wires are attached to the scalp. The electrical activity is measured and compared to that seen in normal children. This test is often normal in children with spina bifida and hydrocephalus. It is most helpful in seizure disorders, but these are rare in children with spina bifida. Your child may be unhappy having the small wires attached to his scalp, but it is not painful.

When Hydrocephalus Needs Treatment

When the head size is growing too rapidly or the ventricles are enlarging too much, treatment will be needed. Safe and relatively simple procedures, such as skull x-rays and a CAT scan, are usually the first steps. Following these an air study (ventriculogram or pneumoencephalogram) may be necessary. These studies will show the size and shape of the ventricles and demonstrate whether communicating or noncommunicating hydrocephalus is present.

If the spinal fluid pressure is excessive, it needs to be relieved surgically. This is done by means of a shunt operation.

The Shunt Operation

A shunt is simply an artificial pathway for the fluid inside the brain or head to be returned to the bloodstream. Many methods for doing this have been devised, but the most common one in use today is a tube that goes from the ventricles to the abdomen. It is called a ventriculo-peritoneal shunt (VP shunt) and is a relatively simple surgical procedure. During surgery an incision is usually made behind and above the right ear. When the hair regrows later, this scar will not be visible. Beneath this incision, a small hole (called a Burr hole) is made through the skull. Through this hole a delicate siliconized plastic tube is placed directly through the brain and into the ventricle. On the outside of the skull this tube is attached to a small valve. The other end of the tubing is placed in an area of the body where the

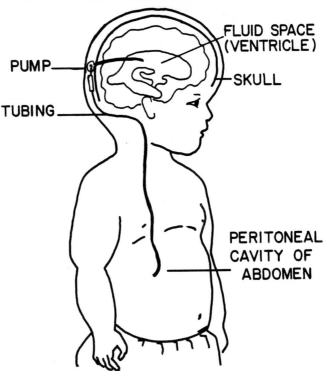

VENTRICULO-PERITONEAL SHUNT

FLUID SPACE (VENTRICLE)

PUMP

SKULL

TUBING

PERITONEAL CAVITY OF ABDOMEN

Figure 13-3.

VENTRICULO–ATRIAL SHUNT

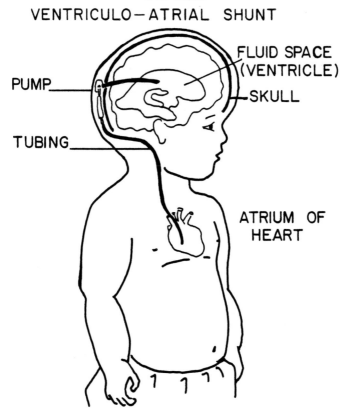

Figure 13-4.

fluid can be absorbed back into the bloodstream. This end is usually put into the abdomen, but in the past it was often placed in the heart (ventriculo-atrial shunt) VA shunt. The tubing is passed under the skin from the head to the abdomen. A separate small incision on the abdomen is necessary in order to properly place the tubing. Many other sites have occasionally been used in the past, but placement in the abdomen seems most successful.

This tube system has valves so that the fluid can flow in only one direction. The flow is from the ventricle to the area for absorption, in this instance the abdomen. These valves are sensitive to pressure and only open when the pressure inside the brain reaches a certain level. This prevents the pressure within the brain from falling too low, as well as getting too high. Two commonly used valves are the Holter and Pudenz.

After the Operation

You will have to be careful handling your child until the incision heals. When healing is complete, the only precaution needed is to avoid banging or bumping the head. The tubing which lies outside the skull can easily be felt under the skin. The valve is usually positioned behind and above the ear on the right side and can be felt, but not easily seen, under the hair. The valve can be pressed without producing pain and this is a useful test to determine how well the shunt system is working. The valve usually collapses under light finger pressure and then refills with fluid. The valve is helpful in determing the location of a blockage if the shunt stops functioning. If the valve does not collapse, then there is an obstruction beyond it. If the valve pumps but fails to refill, then there is a blockage between the ventricle and the valve. Obstructions can result from scar tissue growing around the tubing or occasionally from blood, blood vessels, or brain tissue blocking one end of the tube.

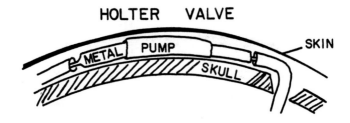

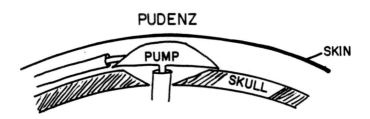

THE TWO COMMON TYPES OF VALVES
WHICH ARE PLACED IN SHUNTS.

Figure 13-5.

Several types of valves are available and the means of testing how well each one functions are different. Some specialists prefer that parents do not pump the valve. If your doctor wants you to check the valve, he will tell you to do so and show you the proper method.

Generally, these drainage systems work very well but new improvements are constantly being devised. As a child grows, the tubing may become shorter in relation to the length of the child's body. This may require that parts of the system be replaced periodically. Often extra tubing is placed in the abdomen so that as growth occurs the tubing will simply be pulled out of the abdomen, but the end will still be in the proper place and the shunt will continue to function. Other methods of solving this problem which growth creates are currently being studied.

What If the Shunt Fails?

If a shunt fails, it usually occurs over several days to weeks. During this time the pressure builds slowly and some of the following signs and symptoms give warning that a re-evaluation and perhaps a revision of the shunt is necessary:

Headache
Irritability
Vomiting
Drowsiness
Swelling around the tubing or pump
Episodes of confusion
Tremors of the hand or eyelids
Progressive loss of consciousness
Sudden episodes of total body rigidity

What Should I Watch for?

Shunts usually work very well. However, there may be occasions when they work only partially or not at all. The response your child will have depends on whether the blockage is partial or complete, and how your child's nervous system reacts to the increased pressure inside the head. A shunt which is only partially functioning may correct itself over time and, therefore, may simply require close observation. At times shunts appear to block and then reopen spontaneously. This can even occur several times and is called an intermittent shunt blockage. A totally nonfunctioning shunt usually requires some type of surgical repair. A period of observation may be required in order to determine which is the case and to make sure that surgery is absolutely necessary. This observation period can be a very upsetting time for parents. Their child may seem very ill, and they may be worried about possible brain damage. During this time they are asked to wait and place faith in their physician's recommendations. Determining the danger of brain damage, and the need for further surgery, is a judgment that your child's physician must make. Unnecessary surgery, especially involving the brain, should be avoided whenever possible.

Other Complications of Shunts

Mechanical failure or simple blockage are the most common problems, but others occasionally occur. A blow to the head, such as a fall, might cause the tubing to split, break, or separate from the valve. A revision or replacement of the shunt would then be needed.

Whenever a foreign object is placed inside the body, it can be a focus of infection. Shunts are foreign to the body and occasionally become infected. When this occurs there is often persistent fever and symptoms similar to those of shunt blockage. In the past when the shunt tubing was placed in the heart, this was a more common problem. The placement of shunts in the abdomen and outside the bloodstream has greatly reduced the frequency of shunt infections. The diagnosis of shunt infection can only be made with certainty by examining the fluid either within the shunt or the ventricle itself. Since the ventricle is only reached by passing a needle through the brain, this is usually avoided and the fluid within the shunt examined. This can be done easily by placing a small needle through the skin and into the shunt valve. Fluid is then removed and examined. Although the technique is simple, there is a danger that the shunt will be damaged by doing this. Should this occur, the shunt would need to be repaired or replaced even if no infection were present. Since there are many more common causes of fever in children, this procedure is reserved for special situations. If an infection of the shunt is identified, then antibiotic treatment is necessary. Usually the shunt is removed until the infection is cured and then it is replaced. The infection may not respond to treatment unless the shunt is removed.

How Long Must the Shunt Remain?

Once a shunt has been placed, it is usually removed or replaced only for a very good reason. Blockage and infection are the two main reasons. If a shunt becomes blocked but the child remains well, surgery would probably not be considered. Partial blockage of a shunt may be difficult to determine, but every effort should be made to avoid unnecessary surgery. Shunts are usually permanent once they have been placed. A shunt should be place only when it is clearly necessary.

CHAPTER 14

THE EYES

YOUR CHILD'S EYES

CHILDREN with spina bifida often have problems with their eyes. Strabismus or a lazy eye, where one eye is looking at an object and the other is turned either inward or outward, is especially frequent in children with spina bifida.

The coordination between the two eyes and the movements of each eye are accomplished by a complicated, delicate array of nervous pathways in the brain and upper spinal cord. If these pathways are not all functioning properly, the eyes do not work together. When strabismus is present, the child sees with only one eye at a time. The brain simply ignores the picture received from the other eye. If the eyes do not see the same thing, then either they take turns seeing (alternating strabismus) or consistently only one eye is used (strabismus of one eye).

Alternating Strabismus

As the child with alternating strabismus looks at you with one eye, the other eye turns in or out. Then, in a split second, he may switch and look at you with the other eye. When this happens, the eye which was originally looking is the one that turns. This alternation of eyes goes on almost constantly, and the child is unaware of any trouble seeing.

Strabismus of One Eye

In this situation, the child always views the object of his interest with one eye and the other eye constantly turns inward or outward. Again, the child is not aware of any vision problem, since his brain simply ignores the image it receives from the eye that is turning. After several weeks or months of the brain's constantly ignoring or suppressing the image of the turning eye, the brain begins to lose the ability to see images from that eye. Blindness develops in this eye even though its nervous pathways are still intact. The eye that turned in or out eventually loses its vision.

What Does the Physician Look for?

The most important responsibility of the physician in caring for a

137

child whose eyes are turned is to know whether or not suppression of the vision in one eye is taking place and whether blindness is developing. It may be very difficult for the physician to be sure how well a child under four or five years of age sees, but every effort must be made to determine this. Examination to detect a possible need for glasses must also be included so that confusion does not arise about the source of any trouble seeing.

Some children with spina bifida do have a defect in the nervous pathways which carry sight from the eye to the brain. Such a defect of the optic nerve is uncommon but may be present at birth. It does not generally respond to treatment. Partial damage to the optic nerve may also occur but does not prevent all vision. It may cause only a slight disability, and it may occur in one eye only. It is important for the physician to know whether or not the poor vision he finds is due to the progressive blindness from suppression of one eye, or whether it was present at birth.

Why Is the Diagnosis So Important?

The reason that it is so important to diagnose the source of progressive blindness is that it can be corrected if it comes from the brain suppressing the image of a turning eye. It is essential that this be corrected at the earliest possible age.

How Is It Corrected?

The most effective method of treating and correcting strabismus from suppression (amblyopia) of the turning eye is by interfering with vision in the good eye. Covering the good eye constantly, using eye drops to interfere with its vision or some form of eye patch are the most frequent methods. This often results in reestablishing coordination between the brain and the deviating eye and good vision may be restored. Unfortunately, the process may take many months. Even when it is successful, it may need to be continued at least part-time for many years.

It is simple for the doctor to recommend patching one eye, but the real responsibility for the success of this treatment rests with the parents. Sometimes parents find it difficult to insist that the child constantly wear the patch. The child may vigorously resist this treatment, since his vision may be reduced to a quarter or tenth of what it would be if he could use his good eye. Therefore, you may need to be very firm and prepare to offer some extra support and attention. You need to understand that the child is undergoing an unpleasant but painless treatment. Success is often achieved, and you will find it most gratifying when you have accomplished something in the end.

When patching is not considered adequate to handle the problem, an operation on the eye muscles can be done by an opthalmologist (eye surgeon). The chances that this surgery will be beneficial are excellent.

Other Eye Problems

While strabismus is the most common disorder in children with spina bifida, there are a number of other eye conditions which can be found. Generally they are related to the fact that children with spina bifida also often have hydrocephalus. Some of these other problems are:

(A) Failure of one eye to turn to the side. This usually affects only one eye. When the child tries to look to the side, the eye on the side he looks toward does not move out, but the other eye turns inward. The eyes look normal except when he tries to look to the side.

(B) Failure of the eyes to look upward. The eyes usually look normal, but trying to look upward the eyes do not move. Sometimes the eyes are even turned down and cannot be elevated into the normal position.

(C) Sometimes pressure within the head from hydrocephalus is transmitted to the eyes and changes can be seen in the back of the eye. Seeing these changes requires looking into the eye with an opthalmoscope. What the doctor sees is swelling of the nerve where it enters the eyeball.

These three eye findings are most frequently seen when pressure within the head is increased. They often precede the more common signs of increased pressure such as vomiting, lethargy and headache. If you notice these conditions occurring, you should contact your physician. They may be indications that a shunt is not working. Occasionally they occur for other reasons, but your physician should evaluate the situation and determine if a specialist should be contacted.

CHAPTER 15

MUSCLES AND BONES

SITTING, STANDING AND MOVING FOR THE CHILD WITH SPINA BIFIDA

MOST children with spina bifida have some muscle paralysis involving their legs and feet. This results in difficulty sitting, standing, moving about and performing other activities that require the use of muscles, joints and bones. Each child with spina bifida is different and has his own set of abilities based in part on the extent of his paralysis.

Whenever one or more muscles are unable to function properly, your child's ability to use that part of his body is lessened. For example, paralysis of back muscles results in difficulty keeping the back firm so that he can sit or stand. Paralysis of leg muscles either prevents the child from using that leg at all or from using it in the same way as other children.

When muscles do not work properly, they do not protect the joints and bones like they should. In time this can lead to problems in the joints or bones themselves. Helping prepare your child to sit, stand, and move about will constitute a large part of his medical care. It is an area that concerns most parents.

How Muscles and Joints Usually Work

Bones are connected by joints and in the legs most of these joints allow for movement. Movement results when a muscle that connects the bones on each side of a joint either tightens or relaxes. Usually at least two muscles cross each joint but sometimes there are many more. The hip joint can move in many ways and there are many muscles that influence its movements.

Muscles are helped by ligaments. Ligaments are strong tissues and act like biological ropes. They connect bones across joints and prevent excess movement at the joint. When they tighten, muscles cause either movement at the joint or stabilizing of the joint. When muscles are not working properly, the joints which they affect are not stable and motion at these joints is not controlled by the child.

140

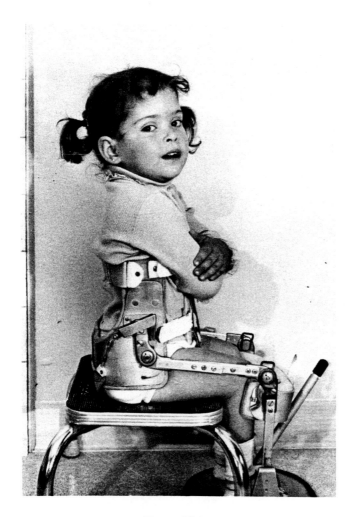

Figure 15-1 a.

The Effect of Paralyzed Muscles

When the muscles and ligaments around a joint tighten so that movement is more limited than normal, it is known as a contracture. Contractures can result from partial or complete paralysis of muscles. The movement may be limited in only one or in several directions. For example, if a child with spina bifida has effective muscles to straighten the knee, but the muscles required to bend it are paralyzed, it may become increasingly difficult to bend the knee, unless the knee

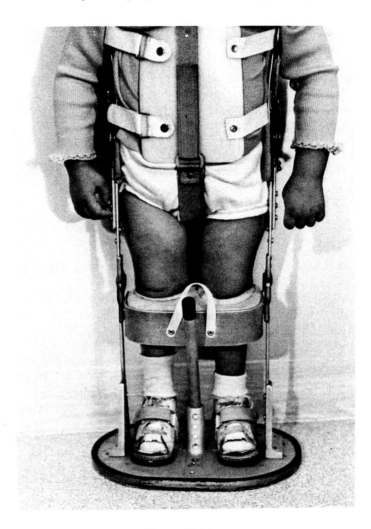

Figure 15-1 b.

is kept flexible by frequent exercises. Contractures usually occur slowly over weeks or months. The same situation can occur at any other joint. The power to turn the foot inward without a balancing power to turn it outward will eventually lead to a stiff foot that is turned inward. Hips which can be bent upward and brought together, but which your child cannot voluntarily separate or straighten, tend to become contracted in a position where they are upward and together. If this position is allowed to persist without stretching exercises in the opposite direction, changes in the bones around the joint may eventually take place. Sometimes it is difficult or impossible for exercises alone to prevent contractures.

The Loss of Skin Feeling

We have been talking about how paralysis prevents muscles from moving and working in the correct way. Other nerve pathways, similar to those which cause muscles to move, carry feelings of touch, pain and other sensations from the skin to the brain. These sensory pathways are also interrupted by some forms of spina bifida. When these pathways are damaged, the child cannot feel in the affected areas.

The loss of feeling for touch, heat, pain and other sensations from the skin can lead to many problems. Sensations such as pain and heat are what tell us that the bath water is too hot, that we have sat too long on one area of skin, that a bone is broken, or many other messages which help us to protect our bodies. This loss of sensation is especially important when the child is in a cast, braces, or has limited independent movement.

Why Is Being Upright and Moving So Important?

Much of the health team's effort is directed toward helping your child be upright and mobile. There are a number of reasons why this is important.

Psychologically being upright offers many advantages. We live in a world where people sit, stand and view each other upright. A child who is looked down upon because of his inability to stand is immediately at a disadvantage. If he is upright, he will be able to see more and begin to interact with others in a new manner. He can begin to exert his own will and, as a result, can view himself more positively. The ability to move about will also improve his self-respect. It will allow him to do some things for himself at times that he can partially choose. This new independence and self-image will also influence how others view him.

These reasons alone would be adequate, but in addition there are medical benefits. In the upright position, gravity helps the kidneys to drain better. This helps prevent urine infections and other kidney problems. Bones and muscles which are not used regularly become weaker. The growing child who does not use his legs develops increasing weakness of the bones. In addition, an important stimulus to normal growth of the legs is the pressure of muscle activity and bearing weight. If the legs do not grow to normal size or strength, they are more easily broken when minor injuries occur. By providing growing bones with the stress of bearing weight, they grow stronger and are not as easily broken.

How Can These Goals Be Accomplished?

Helping the child with spina bifida to be upright and independently mobile requires the efforts of many people. The effort starts at home, where he should be encouraged to use his abilities to the fullest, to exercise and to develop adequate strength in the shoulders and arms. Then with encouragement he can use the braces and other aids which will help him to accomplish these goals.

Many health professionals can assist you, but the central ones helping in this area are the orthopedist, the physical therapist, and the orthotist (bracing specialist).

Besides developing his abilities to the fullest, your child needs to compensate for his disabilities. For example, most children with spina bifida have normal use of their shoulders, arms and hands. The muscles of the arms, hands and shoulders can be strengthened and trained so that they partially compensate for the paralyzed muscles in the lower extremities.

The physical therapist can show you: how to strengthen your child's shoulders and arms; how to stretch muscles so they do not develop contractures; how best to use braces, crutches and other devices; and a variety of other ways to help him increase his skills and utilize his abilities.

Bracing is often able to help children use limbs that are only partially under their control. The orthotist, working with the orthopedist and physical therapist, is responsible for building the many devices which help children accomplish this. He sees that the braces fit correctly and makes the necessary adjustments as the child grows.

When exercises or bracing are not adequate, or when certain other problems occur, surgery may be necessary.

The orthopedist guides and directs exercise programs and bracing and may perform operations to make the bones, joints and muscles work as well as possible. No matter how successful the physical therapy and bracing, surgery may still be needed. Many children who have spina bifida need one or more orthopedic operations.

The Body Areas Where Bones, Muscles or Joints Need Attention

Many children with spina bifida have been helped significantly by this combined approach of exercises, bracing and surgery. A review of the body areas where problems may arise in the child with spina bifida will help you to understand better what may need to be done and how it is accomplished.

The Arms, Hands and Shoulders

The goal with the upper limbs is to strengthen them so they can be used effectively in moving about. Fortunately, children with spina bifida usually have normal upper limbs. Occasionally weakness or tightness of the arms is present.

It is important for the child with paralysis of the legs to have extra strength in the arms so that he can move about with the aid of braces and/or crutches. Because of this, arm strengthening exercises should be started as early as possible.

The Spine

The purpose of the spine is to support the child's trunk and assist in sitting and standing. The backbone or spine is the main bony support for the trunk. It prevents the trunk and head from collapsing when the body is upright. It also protects the nervous tissue of the spinal cord and serves as anchoring points for the muscles which move the trunk, shoulders and hips. The normal spine is straight when viewed from the front; and when seen from the side there are several gentle curves. In the neck (cervical) region, the curve is normally arched to the front (lordotic). In the chest (thoracic) region, it is normally curved back (kyphotic). The lumbar and sacral regions are normally curved forward (lordotic).

Spina bifida occurs when the bony canal of the spinal column is not completely closed. Part of the back of the vertebrae is not present over one or more vertebral levels. In addition, abnormal vertebrae may also occur elsewhere in the spine. These abnormalities are generally changes in shape (hemivertebrae, wedge vertebrae) or unexpected connections between bones (fused vertebrae, congenital bar). Either type of change will result in uneven growth of the bony spine.

As the infant grows, the curves in the spine may change. This may result in a lateral curve of the spine (scoliosis), and/or excessive forward bending (kyphosis), or backward bending (lordosis). Many combinations of these three basic curves are possible. Kyphosis along with scoliosis is common in spina bifida. The kyphosis usually occurs in the low thoracic or lumbar spine. This occurs when the muscles which attach to the back of the spine are absent. It can also happen if the muscles are not active or lie in the wrong position, because the bones are not properly positioned. The bones in the area of the spina bifida are often curved forward and the attached muscles may pull forward and increase this curvature. As a result of growth and muscle action, the spine may gradually bend forward and, thus, when the child sits the chest comes closer to the legs.

Examination of the spine should be performed at regular intervals

THE CHANGES IN BONY SPINE WHICH CAN OCCUR IN CHILDREN WITH SPINA BIFIDA

NORMAL SPINE

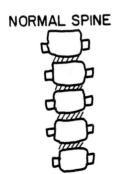

HEMIVERTEBRAE

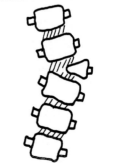

WEDGE VERTEBRAE

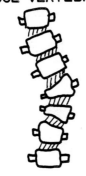

CONGENITAL BAR

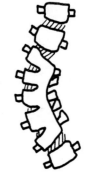

MUTIPLE ANOMALIES

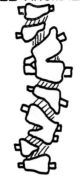

FUSED VERTEBRAE

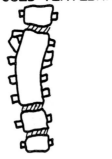

Figure 15-2.

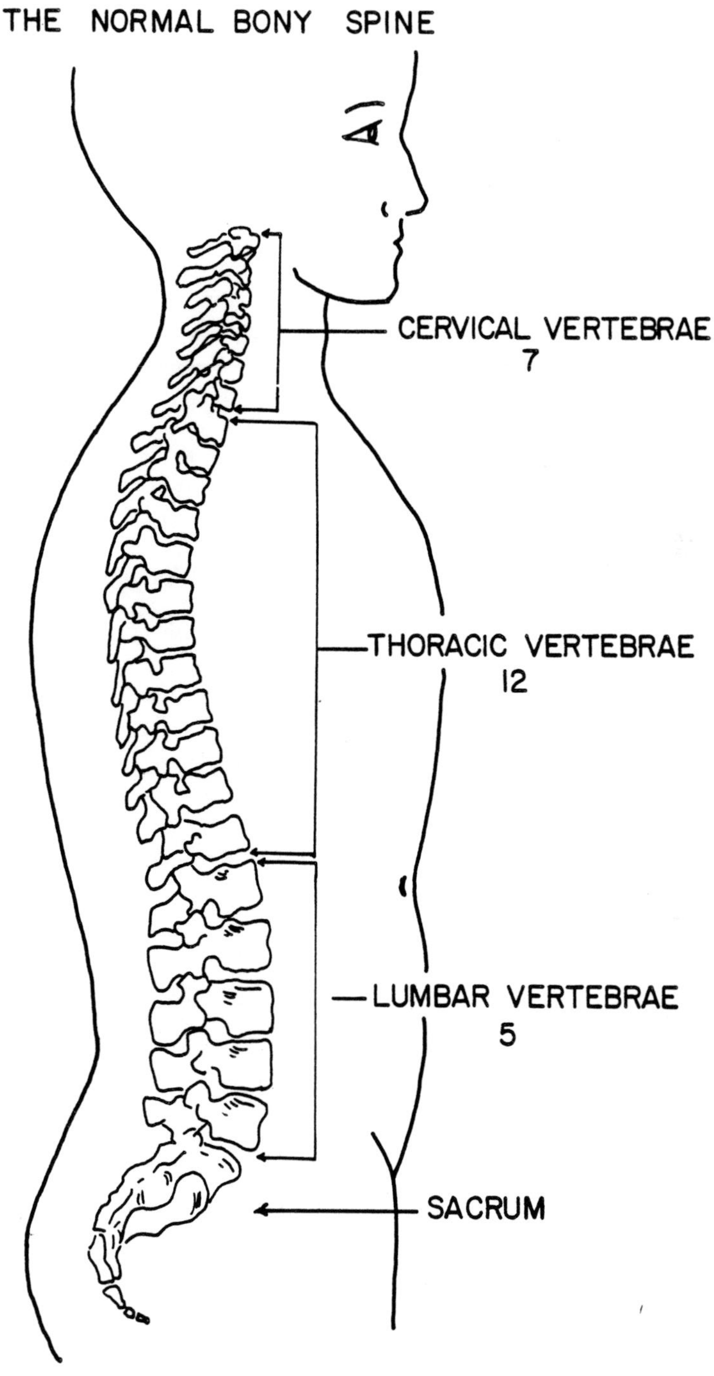

THE NORMAL BONY SPINE

CERVICAL VERTEBRAE
7

THORACIC VERTEBRAE
12

LUMBAR VERTEBRAE
5

SACRUM

Figure 15-3.

SCOLIOSIS

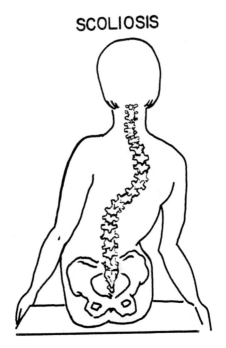

Figure 15-4.

KYPHOSIS

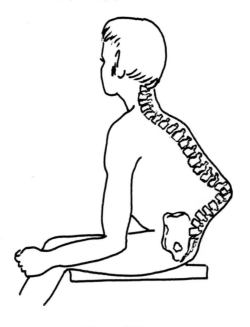

Figure 15-5.

LORDOSIS

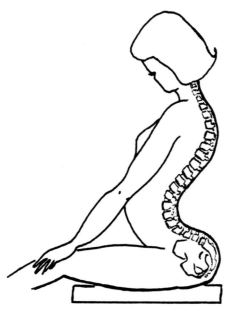

Figure 15-6.

as the child develops, because growth is one of the greatest forces which will cause the abnormal curvatures to increase. The interval between examinations is usually between three and six months. If the spine does not change between exams, then x-rays may not be necessary. However, if a change is detected, x-rays of the spine will be needed to study the pattern of the curvature so that the proper treatment can be recommended.

Once a spinal curve is identified some treatment may be needed. Small curves may need only a spinal or body jacket. This is usually plastic and made from a mold of the child's body. It must be worn most of the time and provides support so that the curve does not increase. Many different types of body braces are also used to prevent or correct spinal curvature, but the most common type is the plastic jacket. You may have heard of the Milwaukee brace which is often used for spinal curves, but this is rarely used for children with spina bifida.

Treatment is intended to provide a more rigid straight spine which will enable your child to sit, stand and move about with the least amount of effort. Surgery may eventually be necessary to correct a curvature or to prevent it from increasing. In this type of surgery the vertebrae are joined together to form a rigid segment in the spine.

This is called a spinal fusion and prevents further growth in that area.

The Hips

The goal with the hips is to keep the head of the thigh bone (femur) in its proper place in the hip socket. This permits movement of the hip for a natural sitting position and allows the child to be upright. Frequently the muscles around the hip become tight if they lack the proper nervous messages. When this happens, stretching exercises in an opposite direction from the tight muscles can lessen or help prevent contractures. These exercises provide some of the activity that would ordinarily be present if the muscles were working correctly. Early bracing also helps counteract the tight muscles and prevents their contracture. Unbalanced muscles pulling on the hip may pull it out of joint (dislocate). When this joint does not work properly, either the hip socket or the upper end of the thigh bone (femur) may not develop normally. As the children grow older some require surgery to change the hip socket or the thigh bone (femur) entering the socket, so the joint can be more stable.

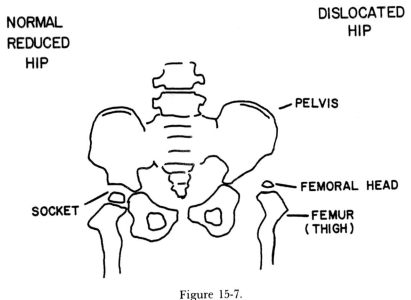

NORMAL
REDUCED
HIP

DISLOCATED
HIP

PELVIS

FEMORAL HEAD

SOCKET

FEMUR
(THIGH)

Figure 15-7.

Dislocation and contractures about the hips may be present at birth. They may also occur later as your child grows and the muscles become stronger. Children who can walk, or are upright in braces, need

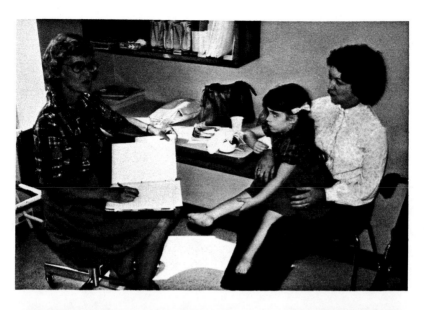

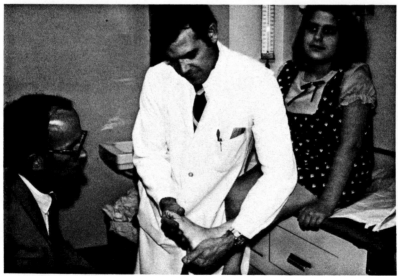

stable hip joints. Those who are not upright may still need their hips treated so that sitting and transferring from the wheelchair will be easier.

The Knees

The goal is to have a stable knee which can bear weight and will bend if the child has adequate muscle use for this. Occasionally, if there are no muscles to bend the knee, but good muscles to straighten it, a condition of "back knee" may occur. Back knee is an awkward and unstable position, but it may be braced. Occasionally a knee comes out of joint and casting, bracing or surgery may be necessary to permit standing and walking.

The Ankles and Feet

The goal is to position the feet so that your child can tolerate shoes and braces for standing and moving without developing pressure sores. The ankle joint is a hinge that allows the foot to move up (dorsiflexion) and down (plantar flexion). There are other joints immediately below the ankle which allow the foot to turn inward (inversion) and outward (eversion). These lower joints also allow some up and down movement.

In some children with spina bifida, deformities such as club foot are present at birth. The degree of muscle imbalance is what usually determines the foot deformity. A child who has a high level of spina bifida may have no control over the muscles to his feet, and his feet may not need correction. However, a low level of spina bifida may affect only certain muscles in the foot. The overpull of some muscles may then cause the foot to turn in, out, up or down. Sometimes the exact muscle imbalance is hard to identify. These are difficult problems to correct. Although such deformities can be temporarily corrected, if the force causing them is not determined and corrected they will occur again.

Nonsurgical treatment of the foot is sometimes possible. This includes plaster casts, bracing in the proper position, and vigorous exercises to stretch tight ligaments and tendons. When needed, there are a number of surgical procedures to help correct the ankle or foot.

Choices in Matters Concerning Mobility

Most parents will find themselves making decisions with the professionals that will influence how their child sits, stands and moves around. As the child matures he may also be involved in these decisions. Most operations on bones, muscles, and joints are not emergencies. There is adequate time for you to discuss and think about such alternatives as waiting for surgery, new bracing or physical therapy. Be sure you understand the information that your doctor and other health professionals provide so that you can make sound decisions.

1. Heel-cord stretching

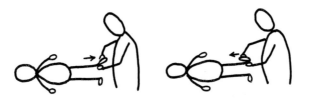

Hold the child's foot by grasping the heel with one hand. Using the palm of your other hand on the bottom of the foot, push the child's foot up towards his shin. Hold this position for a moment and then allow the foot to relax. Repeat 10 times on each foot.

2. Abduction of the hips

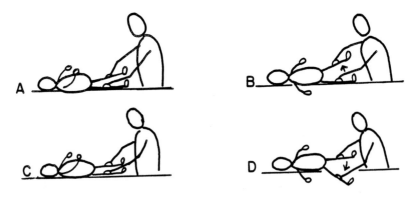

Hold the lefr leg firmly at the knee to prevent it from moving. Grasp the right leg and move it out and away from the left leg as far as possible. Repeat holding the right leg and moving the left leg out to the side. Repeat 10 times.

Figure 15-8 a.

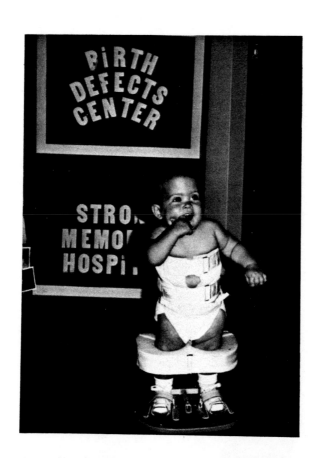

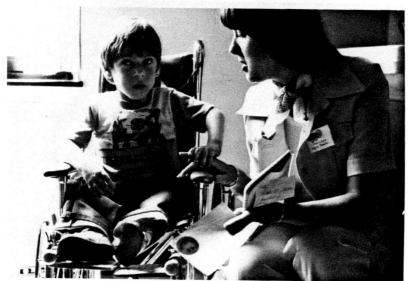

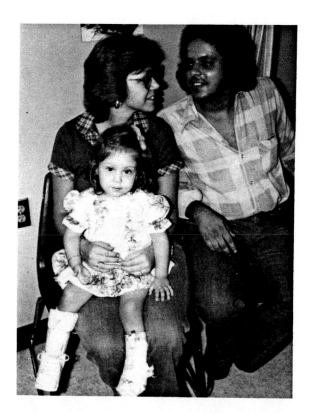

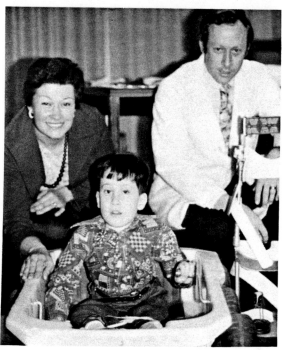

3. Knee extension

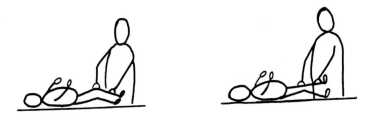

Grasp the leg just above the knee with one hand and at the ankle with the other. Straighten the knee firmly. Hold this position for a few moments and then allow the knee to relax. Repeat 10 times for each knee.

4. Hip flexors and extensors

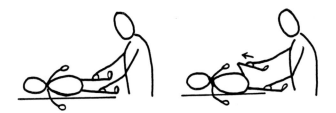

Holding the left leg down, grasp the right leg just below the knee and push the leg towards the child's chest. Repeat this exercise holding the right leg down and pushing the left leg towards the chest. Repeat 10 times on each side.

Figure 15-8 b.

HELPING YOUR CHILD BECOME
MORE MOBILE AND INDEPENDENT

Developing independence requires that your child learn to be self-confident and to do as much as possible for himself. All children with spina bifida are capable of helping themselves a great deal. The major way that you can assist your child to develop his skills is by helping him learn to use all of his abilities to the fullest. Muscles that work well must be strengthened, and devices that assist with mobility and independence must be used to their maximum. Physical and occupational therapy can provide help in many of these areas. An assist from braces (orthotics) is another essential part of this effort.

How Does Physical Therapy Help?

Physical therapy can assist you during many phases of your child's physical development. Some of these phases include different exercises designed to strengthen muscles that will help your child with activities of daily living. Activities of daily living are those things which we all do every day, such as getting out of bed, dressing, eating, toileting and moving about. If your child is having difficulty doing these activities by himself at an appropriate age, a therapist can assist you in developing ways to help your child master these tasks.

Occupational therapy can also be beneficial in helping your child work with his hands such as in dressing or grooming. Again, this type of therapy is designed to help your child actively participate in managing his own daily routine.

How to Encourage Self Care

When your child is old enough to begin dressing, caring for himself in the bathroom, and moving around by himself, then reasonable time must be found for learning these activities. For example, if he is learning to tie his shoes but is too slow to tie them before school each morning, have him practice in the evenings or on Saturday when there is no rush. Then when he learns to tie his shoes quickly enough have *him* do them before school. This type of arrangement will help him learn to do things for himself and yet not be too difficult for the rest of the family. The child with spina bifida may have difficulty doing some dressing and self-care activities by himself, but his need to be independent is as great as any other child's. *Give your child opportunities to do things for himself.*

Types of Exercises

The exercises that the physical therapist will teach you and your child may be to stretch tight muscles or to strengthen weak muscles. Exercises which strengthen weak muscles can usually be done by your child and are termed active. Exercises which stretch tight muscles must usually be done by someone else and are termed passive.

When some of the muscles in the legs work and others do not, the muscles that are working keep pulling and may cause the legs to be pulled out of their normal position. Stretching exercises may prevent this from happening. Sometimes these exercises are effective and sometimes they are not. They help frequently enough that a good effort should be made with them. When they do help, some surgery may be avoided.

Strengthening exercises are done to help the muscles of the arms and legs to be as strong and well balanced as possible. This type of exercise is especially important for your child's arms. When the legs do not function properly the arms become more important and require extra strength. Arm strengthening exercises such as pull-ups should be started as soon as your child can cooperate.

Exercises as Play

Around one year to 18 months of age a child can either understand instructions for exercises or be coaxed into games for this purpose. An example of an arm exercise for a young child would be for him to take your hands while lying on his back and pull up to a sitting position. Most young children enjoy this type of activity and are cooperative for at least short periods of time.

From a very young age, a physical therapist can be helpful in designing stretching and strengthening exercises and practical activities of daily living that are appropriate for your child's age. Your insistence that these activities be practiced at home may be the key difference between a child who progresses steadily toward independence and one who remains dependent. Keep in mind that all children have individual needs, and exercises and tasks should be custom designed for your child and revised periodically as he progresses and grows.

Fitting an Exercise Program into Family Life

Each family must take their child's therapy needs and find a way to fit them into their family life. When the child is very young it is often convenient for parents to do stretching exercises while changing diapers. As he grows older and more activities are added to his program, it is useful to have other family members included at exercise times. Your child may find his exercises are a great deal more fun if he does not feel like he is the only member of the family doing them.

You should follow the exercise program closely but not at the expense of all other family activities. You must remember that each member of the family has their own individual needs. There should be flexibility in the exercise program. If there is a special family activity, do not eliminate that activity but rather find an alternative time for the exercises.

Infant Exercises

During the first year your child will be mastering several motor skills. He must learn to control his body. Mastering these skills will result in the ability to sit, stand, and move about. The following is the usual order that children learn these skills.

1. *Rolling*. After four or five months of age he will begin to push-up on his arms and look at objects around him. As he grows stronger and gains coordination, he will push higher and eventually (and usually accidentally) push so hard that he rolls onto his back. This usually causes great joy for both the parents and the child, and he will repeat this over and over. When the legs are paralyzed this is more difficult to accomplish.

2. *Sitting*. Around six to seven months of age your child's back should be getting stronger. At this point you should begin propping him in a corner of the couch so he can sit by himself. Do not leave him alone, however, since he will not be strong enough to sit long by himself. If he is not able to sit propped in a corner at this stage, speak to your therapist. She will have suggestions on ways to aid your child to sit. If there is any weakness of the back, this task will be more difficult for him.

3. *Belly crawling*. At about seven to eight months he should be rolling in both directions and using this method to reach objects he wants. At this time he may discover that he can pull himself along the floor with his arms while lying on his stomach. This is the beginning step to crawling. If he has not begun this activity, make sure he spends some time each day on his stomach. Take adequate time each day to encourage this activity. Your presence will help him enjoy being on his stomach. Even children with paralysis of the back and lower legs can move about by belly crawling. If a child is unable to crawl, a caster cart or Crawl-a-gator® may be useful to encourage him to explore his environment.

4. *Crawling and coming to sitting*. These two activities occur at about the same time around the ninth or tenth month. You may find him trying to rise on his hands and knees; but if there is leg weakness, this will be difficult. You can help him in his attempts by sitting behind him and supporting his hips and legs. Then place him in a crawl position in order to give him the feeling of that position.

    Most children learn to get to a sitting position by first being up on their hands and knees. For this reason, the child who has difficulty crawling is also likely to have trouble getting to a sitting position by himself. One technique for helping is to have your child roll onto his side and then use his hands to push himself up into a sitting position.

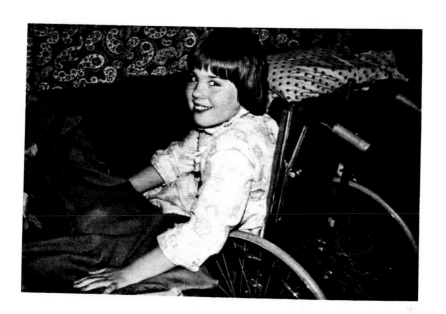

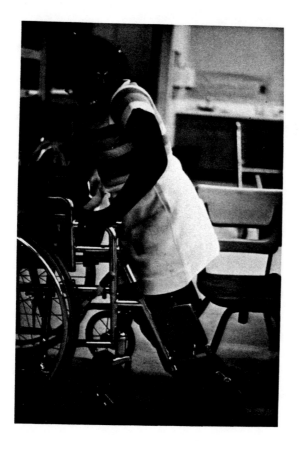

5. *Pulling-up.* Around the age of one year you may see him trying to pull to a standing position on a piece of furniture. If he is unable to pull to a standing position after several weeks of trying, then devices to aid him in standing should be considered.

Again, it is important to remember that each child with spina bifida is an individual and has different abilities. Each child grows and develops at his own rate. The time schedule for the activities that has just been outlined is only a guide and should simply be used as a reminder of how a child can be helped to experience activities that are appropriate for a given age. This outline may also give you an idea of the developmental steps where your therapist may be of help.

Equipment for Sitting

There will be periods of time during your child's day when sitting will be practical. For these occasions one of the following aids may be helpful.

1. *Corner chair.* This is a device to aid the child who is beginning to sit by himself but still needs support. It is constructed with three pieces of wood which form a corner. The seat can be placed on the floor where the child is safe, secure, and able to play with objects placed near him. A small table can be placed in front of him making it easier for him to play with toys. A safety belt can even be added to help him maintain his position.
2. *Caster cart.* This device is a good way to help the child with paralyzed legs to explore his home. This cart, like the corner chair, is built very low to the ground so that he can crawl in and out of it. In addition, he can pick toys and objects up from the floor. The cart is designed with three wheels. Two of these are placed so that the child can reach them with his hands and move the cart in any desired direction. This cart is appropriate for use as soon as the child is interested in pulling himself along the floor or if a child has not begun to crawl by one year. A detachable handle can be fixed to the back so others can push him in the cart.
3. *Wheelchair.* As children grow older and become heavier, it may be necessary to obtain a wheelchair. For many children with spina bifida there will be times when it may not be practical to walk or move about while standing. If he is using crutches and braces to walk, he will be using approximately two to three times the energy to cover the same distance as other persons. For this reason, he may be more comfortable using a wheelchair for long distances.

Wheelchairs come in many sizes and styles, and this is another

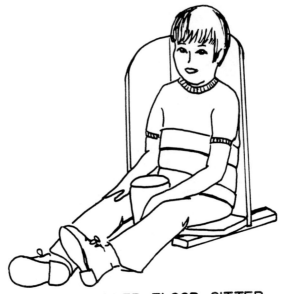

CORNER FLOOR SITTER

Figure 15-9.

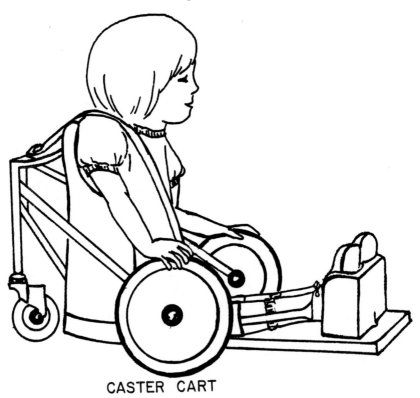

CASTER CART

Figure 15-10.

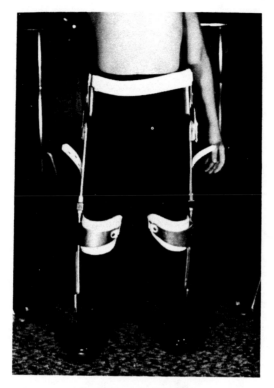

LONG LEG BRACES

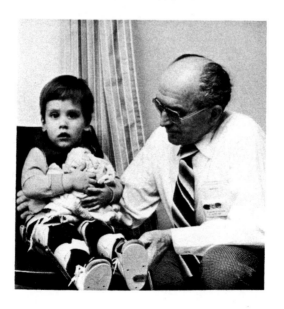

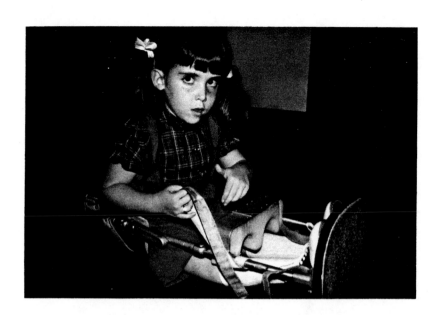

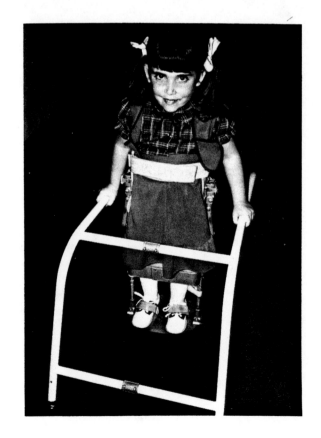

area where your therapist can help because there are many things to consider before any purchase. Some of the most important considerations are your child's height and weight, his rate of growth, and where he will be using the chair. Some wheelchairs are designed for self use while others are not.

Since you are with your child daily, it is important that you tell the therapist when he is learning each of these activities. This will help the therapist update activities on which your child should be working.

BRACES AND DEVICES TO IMPROVE MOBILITY AND SELF-SUFFICIENCY

The Orthotist's Role

Many children need braces or other devices to assist them in their efforts to move about and be self-sufficient. The orthotist's goal is to help your child become independent in his environment. An orthotist constructs, fits and repairs braces or devices that will help your child accomplish this. Skillful bracing can work wonders in helping your child improve his mobility.

Braces

A brace or orthosis is any device which fits a part of the body to provide support. For example, if the muscles around the knee joint cannot keep it straight, then a brace could perform this function and help the child to stand. The brace compensates for the strength the body lacks. Without use of the muscles, the joints of the leg will not *support* the weight of the body. A brace replaces the support so that the child can derive both the physical and psychological benefits of being upright. Braces not only give support at times, but they place various parts of the body in the correct *position* to make mobility possible. They can also be used to prevent contractures.

Braces for the lower limbs are divided into four major groups, depending upon the joints they are assisting. They may support the foot, the ankle, the knee or the hip. Some braces support several joints. The spine can also be supported. A plastic body jacket that is carefully molded to fit the individual child's body is one effective method.

Braces are mechanical devices, and it takes time and training for the child to learn to use them. It is especially difficult for small children because they do not understand their purpose. After a child knows that he can do things better in a brace (sitting, standing, moving around), it often becomes like a piece of clothing. You will need to be firm but kind about using the brace, since children are influenced by their parents' attitudes toward the brace.

Regular check-ups while the child is in the brace are important.

Active children cause wear and tear on the brace parts, and refitting may be needed due to growth. Other physical changes can also make it necessary to adjust the brace. You should check the brace regularly for signs of wear, and be sure the movable metal parts are oiled.

The Parapodium

Since the ability to stand is important at an early age, one of the first types of bracing that may be considered for a young child with spina bifida is the parapodium. This brace is one of the simplest types to put on and to take off. It has one lock on each side at the hip. When locked, it keeps the child in a standing position, but it can be unlocked for comfort and a more natural sitting position. The brace has a large oval baseplate under the feet. This base allows the child to stand without using crutches or other supports. This advantage is important for the young child, since he can then use both hands while standing to play with toys and explore objects.

If your child is fitted with a parapodium, he will need time at first to adjust to it. It is well to place him in the parapodium for short periods of time (15 minutes). This should be done several times a day during the first week. You can then slowly increase the length of time he spends in the parapodium, until he is able to wear the brace most of the day. During those first weeks, it is important to check his skin for any red areas caused by the brace not fitting properly. Red areas that do not go away within 30 minutes after the brace is removed, should be reported and the brace checked for proper fitting.

When your child has adjusted to the feeling of standing, he will need to practice rolling and sitting while wearing the brace. He needs to learn all of the developmental skills while wearing the parapodium. These skills will help him feel comfortable and secure while wearing the brace. In addition, you and your child should both learn the methods of falling safely while in the brace. Falling should be practiced until the child can do it easily. This will reduce the fear of falling. Such fear may slow progress in mobility.

As your child learns this first stage of adjustment, the therapist can provide an appropriate sequence for helping him move around in the parapodium. You can also learn how to help at home. There are several ways to walk in the parapodium, and other skills such as climbing stairs and ramps are useful. During the growing years, periodic visits to the therapist for training suggestions will help you and your child use the brace maximally. Appendix E provides suggestions for effectively using the parapodium.

Other Devices to Assist in Walking

When the time comes for your child to learn to walk, he may need

both bracing and other equipment referred to as "assistive devices."
The following list describes some of these devices and is arranged in
the order they are often used in teaching a child to walk.

1. *Parallel bars.* These are stationary metal bars from six to eight
   feet in length which are usually adjustable in height. They give
   solid support and are useful for the beginning walker. Since
   these bars do not move, their use is limited by their position.
   They are excellent for learning techniques and gaining confidence.
2. *Parallel Pusher* (Parallel Walker). This device is a type of walker
   about three feet long and 18 inches wide. Both its width and
   height can be adjusted. It gives nearly as much support as the
   parallel bars; but it is made of light-weight aluminum, and the
   child can move it with him. It can provide support wherever
   there is room to maneuver it.
3. *H-frame.* This is a pair of crutches, usually of the forearm type,

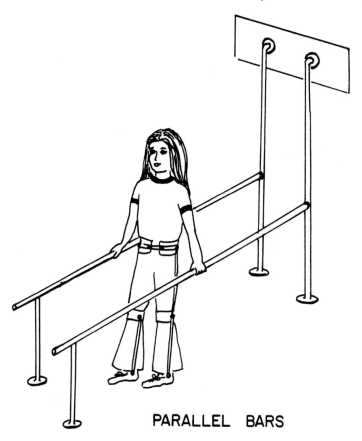

PARALLEL BARS

Figure 15-11.

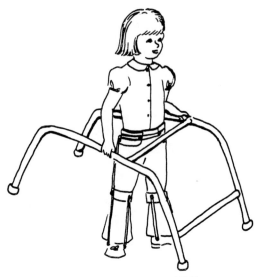

PARALLEL PUSHER

Figure 15-12.

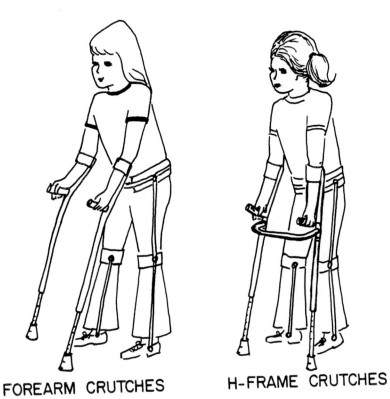

FOREARM CRUTCHES   H-FRAME CRUTCHES

Figure 15-13.

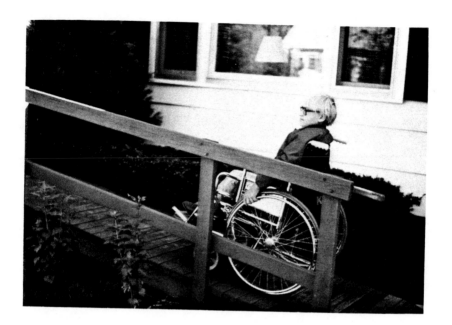

that are held together by a metal bar. These crutches are easier to use than regular crutches. The child must only be concerned with forward-and-backward movement and not with side-to-side movement of the crutches.

4. *Forearm crutches.* When the child is walking well with the H-frame, the bar can be removed and the crutches used individually. Forearm crutches are the most stable type and safest to use for long periods. The individual crutches provide less support than other devices, but there is increased freedom to move in small spaces such as on stairs or ramps. They also take up less space in a car.

5. *Walkers.* There are a variety of devices that are referred to as walkers, and all are similar to the parallel pusher. These walkers are shorter, only 12 to 14 inches long, and do not give as much support as a parallel pusher. They are more readily available, however, and are helpful to children in a parapodium who are learning a swivel-type gait or who have already mastered the

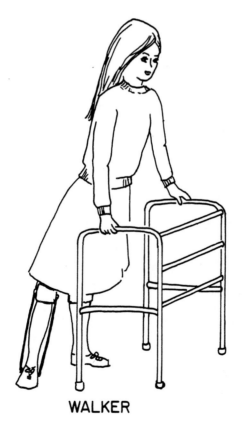

WALKER

Figure 15-14.

swing-gait with a parallel pusher.

Most of the devices described can be obtained from an orthopedic supply shop. If you are not familiar with the supply shops in your area, you may locate them by looking in the yellow pages under orthopedic supplies.

Home Help Aids

There are many aids that can be added to an older home or built into a new home which can make the difference between dependence and independence for your child. If a member of your family is disabled, you should ask some of the following questions before you purchase or build a home.

How Wide Are the Doorways? They should be approximately 36 inches wide to accommodate a wheelchiar.

Is There Any Way to Enter the House Without Going Up or Down Stairs? If not, can a ramp be built with a minimum of expense and difficulty? A ramp inside the garage is best in case the weather is bad.

Is There a Bedroom and Bath on the First Floor? It is important that a child with a disability not have to go upstairs to reach these rooms. To assure independence, the bedroom and bath should be freely accessible. In the long run, the accessibility of these two rooms will save a great deal of the parent's time too. If the house has stairways, they should have at least one railing.

Is the Bathroom Large Enough for a Wheelchair to Enter and Turn Around? If your child uses a wheelchair in the house, he will need this space to be fully independent. A lowered sink without a cabinet, allowing the wheelchair to roll at least partially underneath, is helpful; as is a shower into which the wheelchair can roll.

Can Bars to Assist in Safely Transferring to the Toilet or Bath Be Installed Easily? "Assist bars" can be purchased from an orthopedic supply house and are relatively simple to install. A raised toilet seat is helpful for those who transfer from wheelchair to toilet.

Are the Floorings Practical for Someone in a Wheelchair or Who Has Difficulty Walking? Hardwood floors, tile, kitchen-type carpets, and sculptured carpets are all much easier to manage than are deep shags and plushes and safer than throw rugs.

A practical type of house is a one-floor, ranch style. However, other styles of houses can be adapted.

If you discover practical problems, such as the ones we have been discussing, an occupational or physical therapist may have some suggestions to help you solve the problems. There are countless ways to solve most of the problems of architectural barriers and to help the child with a disability be more independent. Chances are good that your problem has already been solved by someone else.

Activities for Early Brace Wearing

Have your child stand in his brace near a piece of sturdy, solid furniture, such as a couch. This will give him a sense of security. Distract his attention from the natural concern of standing for the first time by helping him play with some of his favorite toys.

Falling in a safe manner should be taught in the first week. The reason this is so important is that learning to fall properly teaches your child he can lean in various directions without falling. This helps him develop a sense of balance in the brace and protects him from accidental falls. It should also help in eliminating his natural fear of falling. Begin teaching him how to fall by sitting in front of him on the floor and asking him to fall into your arms. He will have to rock back and forth to get enough momentum to fall forward. Make a game of this exercise and continue practicing it until you feel your child is no longer afraid. However, do not expect him to conquer his fear the first day.

Skin Checks

It is especially important during the first week to check your child's skin for red marks caused by pressure from the parapodium. If the red marks caused by the brace disappear in 30 minutes, do not worry; but if they do not disappear that quickly, both your child and the brace should be checked. An adjustment to the brace can usually eliminate such red marks. Skin checks should be done regularly, even after the first week, and eventually your child should learn to check his own skin. To help prevent red areas due to rubbing from the bracing, it is a good idea to dress your child in soft, smooth clothes. For instance, tights on a little girl will prevent rubbing of the brace against her legs. Also, a soft T-shirt worn under a body jacket absorbs perspiration and cushions against rubbing. Wrinkles in clothes worn under braces can cause sores, so make sure the clothes worn under a brace are smooth.

Activities After the First Week

If the parapodium is to be useful for walking, it is very important your child feel comfortable in it and that he be able to do as many things in it as out of it. For this reason, teaching your child the following activities while wearing his brace will increase his confidence in the brace and his skill in using it.

Rolling. Your child should be able to roll from his stomach while wearing the brace. This will be necessary later for him to put his own brace on and take it off. Rolling is also essential for him to get to his stomach and push up from the floor to a standing position. So, rolling is very important!

COMING TO SITTING. Your child must be able to sit up in the brace by himself in order to eventually put the brace on and take it off without help. It will be important for him to feel comfortable sitting in the brace during portions of the day, as he will not want to stand for an entire day.

BALANCING GAMES. While your child is standing in the brace, he will need to gain confidence in his ability to stand without assistance and without holding on to anything. One way to develop this skill is to play ball games with him. At first, let him stand in front of a heavy couch and play ball so that he will feel more secure. Then gradually, each time you play ball, try to move him farther away from supportive objects until he is comfortable standing in the center of a room with no assistance.

BELLY CRAWLING. This is the ability to pull himself along the floor on his stomach while wearing the brace. This skill requires strong arms and is a necessary part of learning to get up independently from the floor to a standing position.

Exercises

As your child begins to move about in his parapodium, it will be especially important for his arms to be strong. He will be using his arms for the rest of his life to take over the work of those muscles in his legs which do not function. The following exercises are designed to increase his arm strength:

PUSH-UPS. On stomach — place hands close to shoulders. Lift head and shoulders, and straighten elbows.

CHAIR PUSH-UPS. Sitting — place hands close to hips or on arms of chair. Straighten elbows and lift hips and body.

PULL-UPS. On a bar placed in a doorway, or on a rope, grasp bar or rope and pull body up until weight is being supported by arms alone. If your child is under two years, he can lie on the floor and, by pulling on your arms, pull himself to a sitting position.

What to Expect at Certain Ages

All children mature at their own pace. The following outline is simply a guide to give you an idea of the areas in which you can reasonably work at certain ages.

TWO YEARS OLD. The two-year-old will be able to learn a method of movement called a swivel walk. Some children refer to this gait as a wiggle walk. One way of teaching your child to do this is by first taking his hands in yours, pulling one hand, then the other, and causing the child to move one side of his body forward, then the other. Eventually, the child will pull on your hands rather than you pulling him. At this point, you will need a parallel pusher for him to use as a substitute for your hands. The parallel pusher will give him

Push-ups

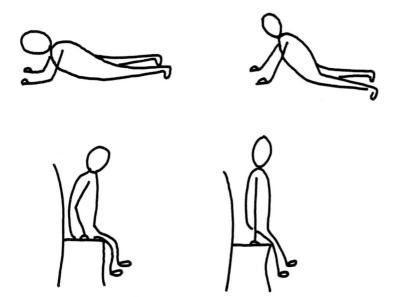

Have child do push-ups from floor or chair each day. Child
should begin with 5 or 6 and build up to 100. The chair
push-up is good for relieving pressure on buttocks and
preventing pressure sores.

Pull-ups

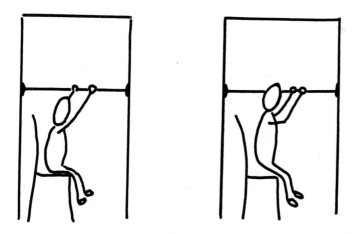

From a rope or bar placed above the child's head, have the
child pull himself up to chin level. This is a very good
exercise to strengthen the arms for walking with crutches.

Figure 15-15.

security and allow him to move anywhere he wishes without your assistance. Some children become sufficiently confident with the swivel gait to do it without any assistance.

A two-year-old can also be expected to master some of the skills required to put on and take off a brace. You should unlock the brace and position it so the footplate (the area in which the feet are placed) is placed against a wall. Your child should then be able to help scoot into the brace and perhaps help fasten some of the straps once he is in the brace. He should also begin unfastening straps to get out of the brace. *This is not to say that a two-year-old can be expected to put on and take off the brace completely, but he can help.*

THREE YEARS OLD. By three years of age, a child can be expected to *begin* moving with what is called a swing-to gait. This gait requires the use of a parallel pusher. The child leans forward on his arms, pushing up, and pulling his body forward in one motion. This type of walk requires strong arms and is one of the reasons for the arm strengthening exercises outlined earlier. It is important that your child develop strong arms at an early age and keep them strong in proportion to his body as he grows. Otherwise, independence is more difficult. *Since the swing-to gait is more difficult than the swivel, do not worry if your child prefers the swivel gait.*

A three-year-old can be expected to manage getting out of a brace by himself if someone helps with the footplate. He should be locking and unlocking the brace with some skill by this age. If he is not, and has been wearing braces for some time, give him more opportunity to do this task on his own. Encourage him to practice during evening hours when the family schedule is not so rushed.

FIVE YEARS OLD. The five-year-old should now be able to lock and unlock his brace as well as put it on and remove it. When the five-year-old has mastered the swing-to gait, he should concentrate on the following activities:

(1) *Getting up from the floor.* This requires balance and arm strength but is very possible. The child who has mastered the previously outlined program of exercises and activities should now be prepared for this task: lying on his stomach on the floor, the child should be able to do a push-up, balance on one hand long enough to reach for a chair or couch, and then pull himself to standing. This task requires considerable practice because it is a complicated skill. However, it is a big forward step in your child's efforts to become independent.

(2) *Transfers.* This general term includes the skills of: moving from a chair to the floor and back; moving in and out of the tub, on and off the toilet, in and out of a car, and to and from bed. All of these tasks require arm strength and balance. Working with a therapist will be very helpful in guiding your child's progress as he masters these tasks.

(3) *Stair climbing.* This task again requires arm strength and

balance. It is best to begin with a demonstration by a therapist and then practice at home.

If your child has been fitted with a brace at a later age (three years of age or older), the general outline of progression is still applicable. Each child must master the activities outlined at his own rate. Some children progress quickly, while others learn at a slower rate.

The parents' role in training a child to become self-sufficient is more influential than any contribution by the therapist. You are the only ones who can be with him a sufficient number of hours each day to direct and encourage his striving for self-sufficiency. With your love and encouragement, your child can achieve amazing things.

ORTHOPEDIC SURGERY

Although the professionals working with your child use exercises, braces and casts, there are some situations where these are not adequate. Surgery may then be necessary. Since surgery is more complex and requires hospitalization, it is reserved for situations where other treatments have not been entirely successful or where it is the best treatment.

When Should Orthopedic Surgery Be Done?

The decision to proceed with surgery is made after the problem has been completely identified and other treatments which have a smaller risk have been considered. Sometimes surgery is needed promptly to prevent a condition from becoming worse, but usually, the timing can be more flexible.

Whether surgery is needed is often a difficult judgment. This is partly because growing children have changing bones. As the skeleton grows, parts of it start as cartilage and gradually harden to form bone (ossify). Cartilage cannot be seen on x-ray and its shape is impossible to determine clearly. As the child grows, problems with bones become easier to see on x-rays. When this occurs, the need for surgery may be recognized. In addition, if muscles pull unequally on bones, the need for surgery may gradually develop.

What Is Done in Orthopedic Surgery?

The surgical procedures for spina bifida are sufficiently complicated that hospitalization and general anesthesia are necessary. This type of surgery cannot be done as an outpatient.

The surgery may be on muscles, tendons or bones. Muscles or tendons can be changed in length, or their attachments transferred, depending upon the child's specific needs. Joints may be put back into the proper position if they are dislocated, and sometimes they are fused solid for greater strength. Twisted or curved bones may sometimes need to be straightened.

Casts Following Surgery

After most orthopedic surgery, the area operated upon must be immobilized until healing has taken place. This is usually accomplished with a cast made of plaster of Paris. Sometimes the cast is cut in half lengthwise and then straps applied so that it can be removed for cleaning and replaced. This is called bivalving.

Casts on the legs and feet are relatively easy to care for, but casts that cover the body and upper legs are more difficult. When the child has poor control over his bladder and bowels, the casts require even more care.

Types of Casts Involving the Body

SPICA CAST. These are used for surgery involving the hips and for some fractures of the thigh bone (femur). There are various sizes and types of spica casts.

(1) *Single hip spica.* This cast covers the trunk up to the lower edge of the chest and includes one leg down to the toes.

(2) *One and a half spica.* This cast is like the single hip spica, but also extends to the knee of the other leg. There may be a bar connecting the cast on the legs to give added support.

(3) *Double spica.* Similar to the other spica casts, but both legs are included down to the toes. A bar connecting the leg casts may add support.

Spica casts are frequently applied in the operating room following hip surgery. Several layers of cotton padding are applied before the plaster. The surgical incision may be covered, but later a window can be cut in the cast over the surgical area if there is any reason to check the incision.

WHAT THE COMMON ORTHOPEDIC OPERATIONS TRY TO ACCOMPLISH

Hips

This is an area of many orthopedic problems during infancy and early childhood. The most common problem is unbalanced muscles around the hip leading to the thigh bone (femur) coming out of the hip joint (dislocation). The following are the common hip operations. Sometimes two or more of these procedures may be done at once.

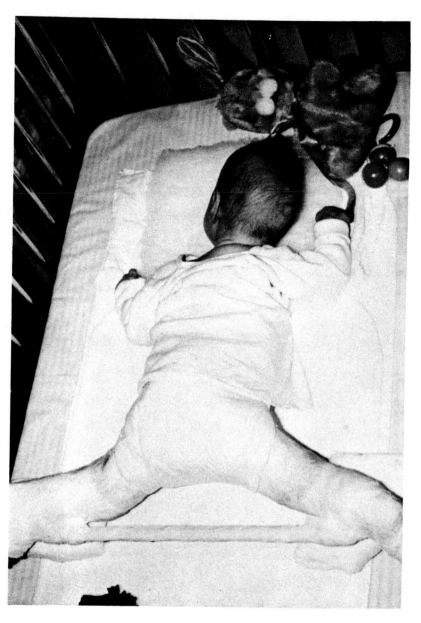

SPECIAL CAST AFTER HIP REPAIR

Reduction of the Hip

(1) *Indications.* When the head or top if the femur is not sitting in the hip socket (dislocation). Movement of the hip is difficult. Ideally, the femur is in the hip socket forming a stable joint which will support the child when he stands.

(2) *What surgery does.* Reducing the hip simply refers to placing the head of the femur into the hip socket. There are two methods.

(a.) *Closed reduction.* Closed reduction means that the bones are moved to the correct position by simply moving them about. This is sometimes possible after the muscles are relaxed by anesthesia. It is done without cutting.

(b.) *Open reduction.* Open reduction means that surgery was necessary to correct the dislocation. The joint was opened and the head of the femur replaced into the hip socket.

(3) *Hospital stay.* About two weeks is required for an open reduction, but only a few days for the closed procedure.

(4) *Cast.* A hip spica is used during the healing period to keep the bones in the proper position.

Flexion Release (Soutter Procedure)

(1) *Indications.* When the muscles in front of the hip are too tight and keep the thigh bent forward. This prevents the child from standing straight.

(2) *What surgery does.* The tight muscles are loosened from their attachment on the femur. An incision is made over the upper thigh.

(3) *Hospital stay.* This usually requires four to eight days.

(4) *Cast.* A cast which keeps the thigh straight at the hip is used for six or more weeks.

Adductor Release

(1) *Indications.* When the hips are tight and the thighs cannot be moved apart or to the side easily. This interferes with useful motion at the hip and may make it difficult to keep your child clean.

(2) *What surgery does.* The muscles that move the thighs together are loosened from their attachment on the inside of the femur. A small incision is made on the inside of the thigh.

(3) *Hospital stay.* This generally takes four to eight days.

(4) *Cast.* A cast which holds the thigh to the side and away from the body is used for six weeks.

Sharrard Procedure

(1) *Indications.* When the muscle which bends the hip forward has no muscle to counterbalance it, the uneven force tends to dislocate the hip.

(2) *What surgery does.* The operation is to prevent dislocation or to hold the femur in the hip socket after it is reduced. It is a difficult operation. The major muscle is released from the thigh, passed backward through a hole in the pelvic bone, and reattached to the femur. The muscle now pulls in a different direction, and this substitutes for the missing muscles which ordinarily would straighten and move the thigh to the side. It also now keeps the femur in the hip joint.

(3) *Hospital stay.* This requires four to twelve days.

(4) *Cast.* A spica cast is worn for at least six weeks.

Osteotomies

(1) *Indications.* An osteotomy is a procedure in which bone is cut. In these operations, a bone is cut into two parts, the parts moved into the desired position, and the bone allowed to heal in a new alignment.

Salter Procedure

(2) *What surgery does.* This is an operation on the bony hip (pelvic bone) to improve the roof of the hip socket. This allows more effective reduction of the hip, and helps prevent dislocation.

(3) *Hospital stay.* The length of hospitalization depends somewhat on other procedures which may be done with this, but it is usually four to eight days.

(4) *Cast.* A spica cast is required for about 10 weeks.

Femoral Procedure

(1) *What surgery does.* This operation is on the upper end of the femur and changes its position so it fits into the hip socket better and will stay in place.

(2) *Hospital stay.* This is usually four to eight days.

(3) *Cast.* A spica cast is worn for at least six weeks.

Knees

Function at the knee joint depends on the amount of muscle paralysis present. The knees may have normal function, no movement, partial movement, or a muscle imbalance.

Flexion Contracture

(1) *Indications.* A contracture is a shortening of a muscle. When the knee is bent and tight muscles prevent straightening it. The knee must be straight to fit braces or a parapodium.

(2) *What surgery does.* This operation loosens the tight muscles behind the knee so the leg can be straightened.

(3) *Hospital stay.* The usual length of hospitalization is four to eight days.

(4) *Cast.* A long leg or spica cast is worn at least six weeks afterwards.

"Back Knee" Surgery

(1) *Indications.* One is when the leg bows backward and the knee is behind its usual position. When this happens, the knee is unable to bend.

(2) *What surgery does.* The attachments of some muscles that normally straighten the knee are moved so that they work to bend or flex the knee instead.

(3) *Hospital stay.* The usual length of hospitalization is four to eight days.

(4) *Cast.* A long leg or spica cast is worn for at least six weeks afterwards.

Foot and Ankle

Heel Cord Lengthening

(1) *Indications.* The large Achilles tendon at the heel acts to pull the heel up. Children with tight muscles, especially if they do not stand and bear weight, may find this tendon has shortened and tightened so that the heel will not touch the ground.

(2) *What surgery does.* The tendon is released and lengthened.

(3) *Hospital stay.* The length of hospitalization is usually four to eight days.

(4) *Cast.* A long leg cast is used at least six weeks. Exercises are needed to keep the tendon from shortening again.

Tendon Release

Just as the heel cord tendon can be lengthened or released, some of the smaller tendons attaching muscles to the foot and toes may be tight and need release and lengthening. This operation is usually performed along with other procedures.

Tendon Transfer

(1) *Indications.* Most muscles moving the foot start in the lower leg and extend down to raise or lower the foot. If some of these muscles are paralyzed, the foot may be stuck in a "heel down, toes up" or a "tip toe, heel up, toes down" position. Sometimes the foot is also twisted in or out.

(2) *What surgery does.* By moving the tendons and attaching them to a new location, their muscles will affect the foot differently. This can help to replace the paralyzed muscles. Transfers are one way to provide the toe push-off which is needed for walking. Transfers are only helpful where at least some of the muscles to the foot are still working.

(3) *Hospital stay.* The usual length of hospitalization is four to eight days.

(4) *Cast.* A short leg cast is used for four to six weeks.

Inner Foot Release

(1) *Indications.* When the front part of the foot turns in. This interferes with walking and can cause sores on the feet.

(2) *What surgery does.* The ligaments and soft tissue connections between the small bones in the foot are released. The foot is then moved into a straight position and allowed to heal. This is often done as part of the repair for a club foot.

(3) *Hospital stay.* The usual length of hospitalization is four to eight days.

(4) *Cast.* A short leg cast is needed for four to six weeks.

Triple Arthrodesis

(1) *Indications.* When foot problems are complicated and the foot is unstable. Often the foot turns in or out so that walking is on one side.

(2) *What surgery does.* Two or three bones may be fused or joined across the small joints within the foot. The ankle joint is still moveable after this operation. This surgery is not done generally until the child reaches his teens.

(3) *Hospital stay.* Hospitalization is from four to eight days.

(4) *Cast.* A short leg cast is usually worn for about 12 weeks.

Things to Know Immediately After Surgery

The length of time in the hospital after surgery varies a great deal. It depends on the type and extent of surgery, complications, and other medical problems which may be present. Even so, there are some situations which are common after most operations.

INTRAVENOUS THERAPY (I.V.'s). Nearly all patients after surgery have an I.V. running. This is continued until the child is able to drink. This is a substitute for fluids withheld on the day of surgery, and a way to administer medication. In some cases, it is continued until the course of medication is finished. The I.V. may need to be changed if the vein becomes red and painful, the needle plugs, or fluid leaks into the skin.

PAIN. Depending on the location and type of surgery, the discomfort will vary. Children are frequently more upset by the restriction created by the I.V. or the cast than by any discomfort resulting from the surgery.

WHEN CAN YOUR CHILD EAT AND DRINK? This is variable. Again, it depends on the type and extent of the surgery, and whether there is vomiting or nausea. Usually eating and drinking will begin the day or evening after surgery.

THE WOUND. The surgical incision is usually not disturbed for about three days. The dressing may be changed earlier, but it is usually not necessary. The stitches are generally removed from 10 days to six weeks after surgery, depending upon the type of surgery and the preference of the physician. Removing the stitches causes very little discomfort, but the idea may be upsetting. The incision should remain dry until it is healed. This means no showers or tub baths. After the stitches have been removed, the incision can be washed unless strips of tape (Steri-strips™) are applied. If Steri-strips are used, the incision must remain dry. Wounds under casts are often not examined until the cast is removed, unless special conditions require it.

THE AMOUNT OF URINE PASSED. This is observed closely after surgery to be sure adequate fluids are being given.

EXERCISE. After the operation, an exercise program may be started. This is especially important if it is a major operation, since other parts of the body must not be neglected while one part is being corrected. These exercises may be passive stretching or active use of various muscles and joints. Breathing exercises are important after certain major surgery, in order to expand the lungs, improve circulation, and prevent complications like pneumonia.

TURNING AND REPOSITIONING. Changing position frequently redistributes the pressure on the skin to different areas and prevents pressure sores from developing. This is especially important after major operations. Changing positions also encourages the lungs to expand and reduces lung complications, helps the kidneys to drain and prevents infection and stones from forming, and makes the child more comfortable.

Your child's other regular needs should also receive attention during any hospitalization. These may include bowel and urinary programs, special diets and skin care. Be certain to discuss your child's unique needs with the hospital staff.

Preventing Fractures

WHY ARE FRACTURES COMMON? When bones are not used, they lose strength and become weak. In children with spina bifida, bones may not grow and develop normally if the legs are paralyzed. Thus fractures may follow minor injury. They often affect the bones in the legs. In addition, a lack of feeling in the legs permits fractures to occur more readily.

Bearing weight should begin soon after surgery to avoid any further weakening of the bones. Weight bearing can be done even in the cast, but you should consult your surgeon before doing this. Usually, fractures occur in the legs at the knee or hip. Redness, warmth, and swelling may be the only signs, and often infection is suspected. An x-ray will show the fracture and clarify the problem.

HOW ARE FRACTURES TREATED? Treatment for a fracture may consist of one or two weeks in a long leg cast, body cast, or simply snug wrapping of the legs to keep them immobile. This may be followed by braces since they offer adequate immobilization. Braces, when worn for this reason, should be worn 24 hours a day except for changing shoes and socks. During changes, you should check for pressure sores. If braces are used, the knees and hips of the brace should be locked all of the time. Standing and walking are needed to prevent further weakening of the bone and to help the fracture to heal. Fractures in children with spina bifida heal as well as in other children and usually require four to six weeks.

Caring for a Child in a Cast

Casts are solid and do not expand when swelling of the foot or leg occurs. If there is too much swelling, the blood circulating in that area may be decreased. This can lead to serious problems such as damage to the skin, muscles or even nerves.

You should check the circulation frequently for the first 24 hours after a cast has been applied and continue to check it until the swelling has subsided. The circulation is checked by looking at the color of the toes or fingers beyond the cast. They should appear nearly normal. When you push on the nail bed of a finger or toe, the area should turn pale; and when pressure is released, color should return quickly. A slow return of color indicates a sluggish circulation. The skin beyond the cast should feel warm and be only a little swollen. The toes beyond the cast can be compared to the toes on the other foot.

Movement of a limb is usually checked by asking if the child can move his foot. In children with spina bifida, this may not be possible,

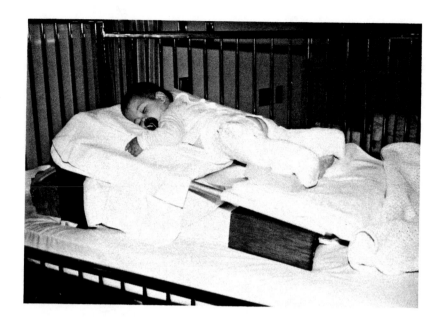

Bradford Frame.

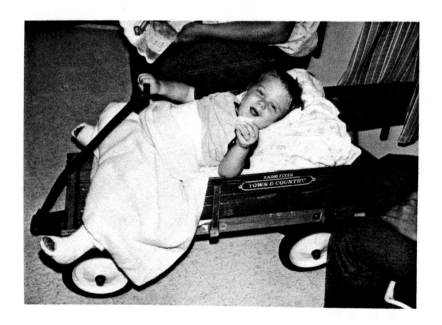

so how the skin looks and feels is especially important.

Discomfort is another sign, but, again, children with spina bifida who lack feeling do not recognize any pain. Deciding what is causing the discomfort may be difficult and young children who are not able to feel may simply be fussy or have a fever.

You should elevate the operative or injured area *higher* than the heart. This will help to prevent swelling, as will cooling the area with ice packs.

The skin around the edges of the cast needs special care to prevent irritation. Tape covering the rough plaster edges of the cast is helpful. You should wash and dry the skin around the cast, and apply powder sparingly around the cast edges. A small amount of powder on your fingertips can be placed under the cast edges as well.

When you move a child who is in a cast, be careful of the toes since they may not be protected and can be jammed into the bed. Be particularly watchful of the toes when your child is resting on his stomach.

Staining of a cast from blood or tissue fluids may happen if the cast is applied immediately after surgery. A wet cast absorbs fluid from the incision, and a certain amount of staining is expected. If any new staining occurs after you return home, you should call your surgeon. This may signal an underlying problem, such as a wound infection or a pressure sore. An unusual odor coming from the cast may also be significant and should be reported to the surgeon.

You should check the cast daily for areas of softening. Softening can occur when repeated pressure is applied to one area, such as hitting the crib with a foot. If this occurs, the cast may need added plaster reinforcement. You should be careful to keep the cast dry, since water will soften it. If the cast appears to be slipping off, you should notify your doctor also.

Cast Checks — What to Look for:

Circulation beyond cast
Movement beyond cast
Discomfort or pain
Skin irritation at edges of cast

Staining of cast
Softening of cast
Slipping of cast

Special Guidelines for a Spica Cast

The spica cast covers the body and hips and is easily soiled by urine and stool. This makes care of this cast difficult, especially in the young child or the child with spina bifida.

You can protect the cast by lining the edges in the groin and buttocks area with plastic. Tuck the plastic under the edge of the cast, fold it back over the cast, and tape it in place. Change the plastic three times during the daytime, or whenever it becomes soiled or wet. Moisture accumulates under the plastic and frequent changes will help prevent skin irritation and keep the cast dry. This is particularly important; because a wet cast is irritating to the skin, can lead to skin sores, and may develop an unpleasant odor.

Disposable diapers work well. You can try to place the plastic between the skin and the cast by tucking the edge of the diaper inside the cast. If your child does not need diapers, place plastic around the groin and buttocks area only when using the bedpan. If the cast becomes soiled, wipe it off with a damp cloth and a little household cleaner.

You should inspect the skin carefully twice a day. A flashlight will help you see the skin under the cast. Press the flesh away from the cast and shine the light under the cast. Clean the skin with soap and water. Dry it thoroughly and then apply powder or cornstarch to the skin. This should be done each time the plastic is changed. When using powder under the cast, apply a little to your fingertips then rub onto the skin.

Blowing cool air with a hair dryer under the cast relieves itching and irritation. A vacuum cleaner is also cooling and removes crumbs from under the cast.

Change your child's position frequently. Turn him every two hours during the day and onto his stomach at least four times a day. When he is turned onto the side, prop pillows under his upper leg. When turning him onto his stomach, it is easier to turn him toward the leg which is in a cast. If the position of the casted leg prevents you from doing this, you may have to turn him toward the other side. Place pads under his feet when he is on his abdomen, so that his toes do not press against the mattress.

Helpful Hints

A wagon is a convenient way of moving a child in a large cast around the house. If he is too large for a wagon, a chaise lounge can be used. A platform with wheels under it, similar to a large skateboard, is another way. The child can be placed on his tummy and use his arms to push himself about.

The Bradford frame is recommended for a child who is not toilet trained and in a spica cast. (See Appendix "C" for directions on how to make one.)

Smaller and more frequent meals may be needed if the cast covers his stomach. Fluids should be encouraged. You should watch for signs of constipation and use a laxative if necessary.

It is a challenge to keep a child stimulated and entertained when he is immobilized in a cast for a lengthy period. The restrictions of a cast are likely to be highly frustrating for him, and he will need outlets through play activities. A bedtray is helpful to hold toys. Encour-

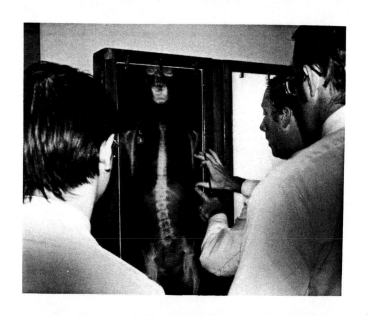

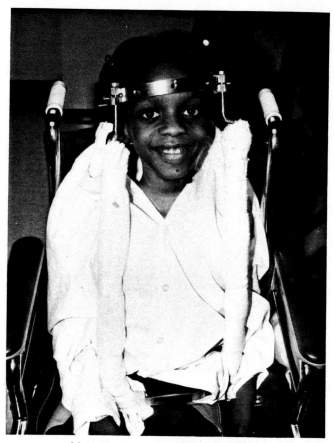

HALO-PELVIC TRACTION

aging him to discuss his care may help him feel better about himself and what is happening to him.

CORRECTING THE CURVED SPINE

Some children with spina bifida develop a curvature of the spine. This usually occurs in the children with larger, higher, or more complex forms of spina bifida where there is extensive paralysis of the back muscles and sitting is more difficult. In these children, and occasionally in those with simpler forms of spina bifida, abnormalities of other parts of the bony spine can also lead to curvature.

Curvature of the spine can interfere with sitting, moving about, and if it is severe enough, with proper heart and lung function. Correction of a severe spinal curvature is difficult, and early treatment when a spinal curve is worsening is considered best. Treatment of spinal curves is complex, but the following is one approach to this problem. Other methods to correct spinal curvature may be equally good or vary in details, but the general principles should be similar.

An initial step in correcting the spinal curve is to straighten the spine, as much as possible, without surgery. This may be done either by traction or casts. Following this, surgery can complete the process of straightening and make the spine rigid. When surgery is performed, it stops growth in those areas affected by the operation.

Casts for the Spine

The localizer cast is often used. This cast comes in various styles and is usually reserved for children who have normal sensation over their entire trunk. The cast starts under the chin and includes the back of the head. It can extend to just above the knees or stop at the hips, depending upon the individual situation. The cast usually has a window cut out over the chest and perhaps over other areas which may need to be viewed occasionally.

The special feature of the localizer cast is that it is applied during traction to straighten the back. This way the cast holds the child's spine as straight as possible. Further correction of the spinal curvature is then obtained by mechanical pressure from the cast. A hinge is placed on one side of the cast and a turnbuckle (a mechanical device which spreads the cast) on the other side. Over several days, the turnbuckle is gradually opened to separate the cast parts, and this pressure straightens the spinal curvature even more. Complete straightening of the spine may not be possible with this method, but most curves can be improved. Wearing this cast is not especially uncomfortable.

The localizer cast is applied on a special table. Before being placed on the table, two layers of stockinette cloth are put over the body to act as padding under the cast. The face is also covered except for a breathing hole, but this part is removed after the cast is applied. Once on the table, traction is applied under the chin, back of the head and to the pelvis. Local pressure is also applied to the trunk to further correct the curvature of the spine. During traction, first a layer of cotton padding, then felt, and then plaster is applied. While the plaster is hardening and being trimmed around the face and arms, the traction is removed. It takes 60 to 80 minutes to apply the cast. This includes trimming the edges, cutting windows and making it comfortable. Sedation or anesthesia is not required for this procedure if the child can cooperate. The procedure is not painful.

After returning to his bed, a cast drying light will be applied for about 24 hours. While the plaster is setting, it feels warm, but later, as it dries, it becomes cool and damp. The drying light helps to keep the child warm.

Traction for the Spine

If a localizer cast cannot be used, traction may be applied in other ways. Halo-Pelvic traction is the most common. In this type of traction, a metal band circles the head and is held in place by metal pins. When in place, it resembles a halo. The pins which hold the halo in place are fastened to the outer bone of the skull. This can often be done with only local anesthesia. In addition to the halo, a second larger hoop is attached around the hips. The pins for this hoop go into the pelvic bones. The halo around the head and the hoop around the pelvis are then connected by four metal rods which each have a turnbuckle. These metal rods are slowly opened or lengthened to correct the spinal curve. A spinal fusion may be done while the child is still wearing the halo traction. This type of traction is also used to keep the spine in the correct position and prevent movement after certain types of surgery.

Although the halo-pelvic traction looks like it might be painful, it is generally comfortable after one or two days. The pins in the head may cause a headache in the first day or two, but then this disappears. The pins in the pelvis are generally painless, since most children with spina bifida who need such traction have no feeling in this area. If feeling is present where the pins are placed, any discomfort usually disappears after four or five days.

The pin sites need to be cleaned with hydrogen peroxide and painted with Betadine® twice a day. The pelvic pins will require dressings around the pins after they are cleaned. If the child has an ileal loop, great care must be taken to prevent urine from draining into one of the pelvic pin sites when the bag is changed. The hair can be washed weekly even with the pins in the head. Pressure must be avoided on the pin sites. This means that turning or moving the child must be done by holding the child rather than using the bars as handles. Padding may be needed around the metal rods in back to prevent pressure over the ribs and the backbone.

Surgery for the Spine (Fusion)

After the curvature of the spine has been corrected as much as possible by casts or traction, surgery may be done. Spinal fusion involves removal of the outer layer of spinal bones in order to expose the soft interior part. Small strips of bone are then taken from other parts of the child's body (usually the pelvis) and grafted to the spine. Sometimes a family member will be asked to donate a bone if the child is small and does not have enough for the bone graft. Occasionally, bone is used which has been obtained from other patients and stored in a freezer at a very low temperature. This bone graft serves as a framework upon which the body builds new bone. As new bone is built, the adjacent bones are fused or joined together. Although the grafted bone dies, it is essential for the stabilizing effect of the spinal fusion.

Spinal Surgery Requires Two Operations

For children with curvature from spina bifida, it is necessary to operate on and fuse the spine from both the back and front sides. Two surgical procedures are necessary, because it is a difficult operation due to the absence of part of the spinal bones and because of the need to operate on both the front and back of the spine.

Common Surgical Procedures for the Different Spine Problems

SCOLIOSIS: Surgery is performed from the back first (posterior approach). A metal rod (Harrington rod) is inserted to help hold the spine while the grafted bones join together in the weeks after the surgery. The Harrington rod is attached to the spinal bones with special hooks. Once inserted, the rod may be tightened to straighten the spine. After the back wound is healed, the spine is then fused in front (anterior approach). Following surgery, a one-piece body cast, a two-piece turtle shell-like cast, or a halo-pelvic hoop are used to hold the spine in the correct position while healing occurs.

SCOLIOSIS WITH LORDOSIS: To correct this problem, both an anterior fusion with Dwyer instrumentation and, later a posterior fusion, are necessary. The anterior approach is done first. The Dwyer apparatus consists of a cable system which is fixed to multiple spinal bones. Correction of the curve is achieved and maintained by tightening the cable. Severe curves may be corrected using this procedure. After the anterior incision has healed, the spine is fused through a posterior approach. After surgery, immobilization is generally provided by a two-piece, turtle shell-like cast. Later a plaster or plastic body jacket is used in the sitting position until healing is complete.

KYPHOSIS WITH OR WITHOUT SCOLIOSIS: Kyphosis must be treated surgically, and it is best to do this early before it begins to increase in severity. This is usually before the age of five years. Once a severe bone deformity is present, extensive surgery is required and there is a greater possibility of complications.

SMALL KYPHOTIC CURVES — AGE 3-5 YEARS: Two surgical procedures are necessary. The first is a posterior spine fusion with Harrington compression rods in the spine. The second stage is fusion of the anterior spine using bone grafts to support the vertebrae in the front. Postoperatively, the child is immobilized in plaster shells or a halo-pelvic hoop until the fusion is mature. This usually takes three to six months. After the cast is removed, protection of the fused area is provided by a plastic body jacket in which the child can sit up.

HARRINGTON   PROCEDURE

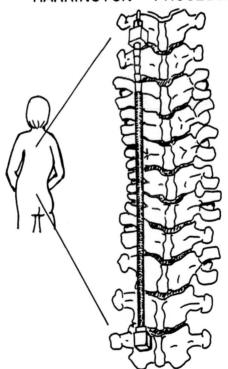

SEEN FROM BACK OF SPINE

Figure 15-16.

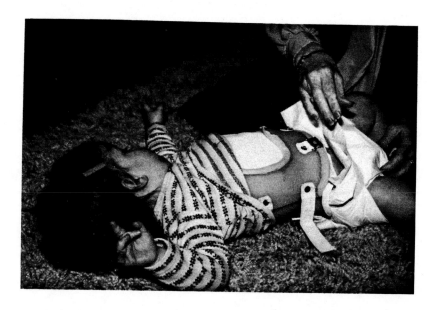

PLASTIC BODY JACKET

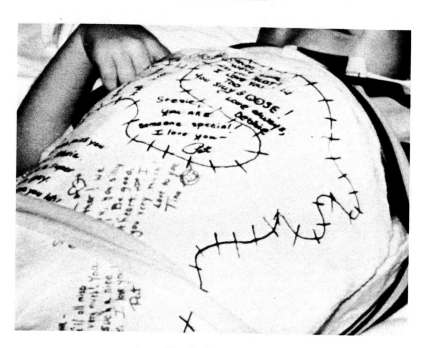

Turtle Shell Cast.

DWYER PROCEDURE

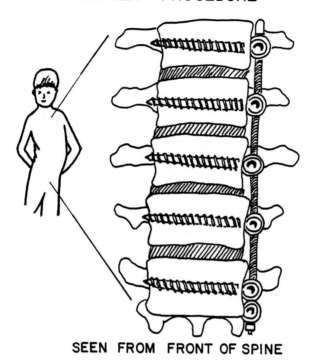

SEEN FROM FRONT OF SPINE

Figure 15-17.

MODERATE KYPHOTIC CURVES — AGE 4-7 YEARS: The procedure is the same as for the small curves, but more correction is required. Part of the vertebrae at the angle of the curve may have to be removed in order to obtain correction. Anterior and posterior surgery are both necessary. After surgery, immobilization and protection of the bone graft are needed for three to six months.

SEVERE KYPHOTIC CURVES — ABOVE AGE 6 YEARS: Severe kyphosis can occur if surgery is not performed at an early age. Kyphotic curves in patients with spina bifida progress slowly, but relentlessly, unless surgical stabilization is performed. When severe kyphosis is present, up to two and one-half vertebra may have to be removed.

With severe kyphosis, the fusion may fail, and a pseudoarthrosis (a false joint) develops in the spine. This causes the spine to bend where it should be straight and to be unstable. In such cases, it may be necessary to operate several times in order to obtain a solid fusion. The length of immobilization after surgery is also longer in such instances, and may approach a year. Protection in a plastic body jacket, until full growth has been attained, usually provides the best chance for success.

Children with severe kyphosis are generally older and thus larger in size. This makes it more difficult to correct the curvature and immobilize the spine. Caring for such a child postoperatively at home may be especially difficult due to the size of the child, the plaster shells, and the length of time immobilization is needed.

Can Spinal Fusion Fail?

Correction of curvature and spinal fusion may not always be successful. Failure can result from the bones not fusing, the graft bending due to growth, the formation of a false joint, or infection. In most spinal operations, several vertebrae are fused simultaneously; but if the fusion fails in only one spot, then a false joint may occur. Another operation would then be needed to repair and fuse the defective area. Why a false joint occurs is not completely understood. Some causative factors may be failure to have adequate external immobilization, too little bone used in the graft, or the occurrence of infection. The success of fusion in children with spina bifida has been greatly improved by doing the surgery both in front and in back of the spinal column. If a posterior fusion alone is performed, the rate of false joint formation is 50 percent or more. The risk of forming false joints in some children necessitates long-term protection of the back by plaster or a plastic body jacket. Sometimes, the older child needs to wear a Milwaukee brace.

When infection does occur at the operative site, the surgery may still be successful. However, infection does usually prolong treatment. If the area of fusion becomes infected, then surgical drainage and treatment with large doses of antibiotics may be needed. After the infection is controlled, some form of skin coverage may be necessary to close the raw clean wound which has probably separated after the surgical drainage.

In summary, spine curves can lead to severe deformities which make aggressive surgical management necessary in order to provide stable support for the trunk. Sitting, ambulating and transferring are all improved when a stable spine is present. A large number of children with spina bifida will require a spinal fusion to enable them to achieve more independence.

Preparing for Anterior or Posterior Spinal Fusion

Preoperative preparation includes an age appropriate explanation to your child of what is to come (see hospitalization). He will probably receive chest and back scrubs to make the skin especially clean and lessen the chances of a wound infection after the operation. Your child may also receive instruction in breathing and coughing exercises. These exercises will help him later to avoid lung problems which may occur if he does not expand his lungs adequately.

What You and Your Child Can Expect After Surgery

You can expect the operation to be lengthy. It generally requires four to six hours for anterior surgery and three to five hours for posterior surgery. After about two hours more in a special recovery room, your child will be transferred to the Intensive Care Unit for one or two days of close observation before he returns to his regular unit. These general guidelines may be modified depending on your child's individual needs, your physician's ideas, and the practices of your local hospital.

After anterior spinal surgery, your child will receive oxygen either through a mask over his face or through a tube in his "trachea or windpipe" (endotracheal tube). The endotracheal tube is inserted directly into the airway before surgery, after he has been put to sleep. When this tube is connected to a mechanical respirator, it breathes for your child and maintains the proper balance of pressure and exchange of oxygen and carbon dioxide in the lungs. Oxygen may not be needed after posterior spinal surgery.

After anterior spinal surgery, your child will also have a chest tube. This is a tube that lies in the space between the lung and the chest wall. This tube allows drainage of any fluid that may accumulate in the space surrounding the lungs. It will be removed when there is no more drainage. Removing the tube is not a painful procedure and is usually done two to three days after surgery.

In both anterior and posterior spinal surgery, two intravenous (I.V.) lines will be running. One is for medications and to maintain an adequate fluid intake, and the other is to measure the central venous pressure (C.V.P.). The central venous pressure reading, along with the blood pressure and pulse, enables the surgical team to monitor your child's fluid balance more accurately. This is especially important if any complications should arise. The I.V. is generally needed for at least five days. There may also be a third tube in one of the arteries. This arterial line is used during surgery and recovery to monitor heart and lung function closely.

For a few days with both types of surgery, your child will have a tube which passes through the nose into the stomach (nasogastric tube). The purpose of the tube is to empty the stomach and prevent vomiting until the normal intestinal function resumes. Your child may complain about how the tube feels and find it annoying, but it is necessary.

Some children require that a catheter remain in their bladder for a few days in order to prevent an excessive accumulation of urine. Children on an intermittent self-catheterization program can continue, but the nurses will need to perform the catheterization using sterile rather than clean methods.

Frequent changes of body position are necessary even in the early days following surgery. The skin must be carefully observed for signs of pressure sores.

Heart function will be followed by using a cardiac monitor. The monitor is connected to your child by means of adhesive discs. This causes no discomfort.

Frequently, a blood transfusion is needed one or two days after surgery in order to replace blood lost during the operation. The blood can be administered through the I.V. that is already running.

When your child's intestinal function resumes after the normal slowdown following surgery, he will be encouraged to drink fluids. If he is able to tolerate fluids well, then the nasogastric tube may be removed and solid food begun.

It is common for children to have an elevated temperature in the first few days following spinal surgery. It is the body's response to the manipulation of the surgery and does not necessarily indicate an infection.

Your child will experience pain from the surgery and will be medicated to be kept comfortable. The need for pain medication should gradually subside with each passing day. The dressing over the surgical incision is usually changed from three to five days after surgery and the sutures removed in ten to fourteen days.

Guidelines for Care After the Acute Stage

The type of immobilization following surgery will vary with each child. The localizer cast, halo-pelvic hoop, and plaster shells are the three basic types. We have already discussed the localizer cast and halo-pelvic hoop. The plaster shells are discussed below.

TWO-PIECE TURTLE-LIKE PLASTER SHELLS. These plaster shells may be custom-molded prior to surgery, if the spine is simply being fused but not straightened or changed in shape. When the spine is being straightened, then the shells are made after surgery in the operating room.

The shells are made of plaster of Paris. First, stretchable cotton material (called stockinette) is cut and placed over the child. Then, felt is cut and molded to the contour of the child so there are no wrinkles or lumps. Next, several layers of wet plaster strips are placed over the felt and molded over the child. The shell for the back is made first, and then the shell for the front. Frequently the shells are lined with artificial sheep skin which can be washed and dried easily. This makes a softer surface and is useful in special cases where skin breakdown may be a problem.

The two shells are strapped together around the child when turning him onto his abdomen or back in a log-like fashion. Care must be taken to protect the legs and arms during turning. With the shells, the child can also be positioned on one side by propping a pillow or blanket roll behind the shell.

Turning

Frequently, the shells are used with the wedge turning frame (Stryker frame). This is a special bed that allows a child to be turned from front to back while keeping the back straight during the turn. Care performed on a turning frame makes frequent changes of position easier. This frame is particularly helpful when the child is older and of large size. Generally, the children are turned every two to four hours during the day whether in the shells, localizer or halo hoop. Without the Stryker frame, the children are simply turned in a regular bed in a log-like fashion. This experience can be frightening, and it is helpful to place the child in the frame and demonstrate the turning several times before surgery.

To Turn with Shells. Apply front shell and strap them together. Pull the child to the edge of the bed. Place one or two pillows so that when he is turned a pillow will be under his chest. Place his arms overhead if possible and support his legs so that they do not twist. Alternately, it may be necessary to put one arm straight down and roll over it. Turn him onto the pillows. The head will need support by another pillow. The legs should rest on pillows so that the toes are not jammed into the mattress. The back shell can then be removed.

To Turn in Localizer. This depends on the size of your child. In order to turn a teenager in a localizer, turn him crosswise in bed, and support his head with the head strap. Then turn him onto his stomach while supporting his legs on a table with a pillow. When turning, his arms should be held over his head to prevent them from getting crushed by the cast. When on his side, pillows can be used to maintain balance.

To Turn in Halo Hoop. Move the child's body. *Do not use the bars for turning.* Lying on the abdomen is generally not too uncomfortable in the halo hoop, since he cannot turn his head to the side. Again, pillows can be used so he can lie on one side.

Using the Bedpan. Turn your child on his side. Place plastic under the cast or shells and around the cast edges in the buttocks area. Place the bedpan under him and roll him onto it. Elevate the head of the bed slightly. Be sure the stool does not creep upward towards the pins in the pelvic hoop. To remove the pan again, roll your child onto his side. Remove the pan and plastic, then clean and dry the skin thoroughly.

Baths. Bathing will need to be done using a washcloth and being careful not to get water onto the plaster cast or shells.

SHAMPOO. Position your child crosswise on the bed and, if possible, on his abdomen. His head may extend over a sink if the bed is moveable. Otherwise, a shampoo tray can be used. He can rest his head over the shampoo tray and water can be poured over it. The water drains out of the tray into a basin below. You can probably devise other individual arrangements with plastic, basins or pitchers.

DIET. Maintain a balanced diet. If your child is in a localizer cast, he may need to eat smaller amounts more frequently in order to avoid abdominal discomfort due to the cast. Try not to let your child gain or lose weight. A weight change would alter the fit of the cast. Adequate fluids are essential to maintain good kidney function, and both fluids and roughage are needed to prevent constipation.

CHAPTER 16

BOWEL CARE

Bowel Control is Possible

BOWEL control is now possible for most children with spina bifida. Although children with spina bifida cannot learn to control their bowels easily, such control can be gained by the use of regular toilet habits, diet and medication. This control takes time to achieve and requires a consistent effort on the part of both parents and child.

Although this goal is not an easy one to attain, the rewards are very large. Your child will develop a greater feeling of independence and control over his body and pride in both his achievement and his ability to satisfy your expectations. Your reward will be seeing your child succeed. Being free of this task should enable you to devote this time to other pursuits.

How the Normal Bowels Work

Knowing how the bowel normally works will help you understand the program for bowel control. The large intestine is the last portion of the intestines. It functions to absorb minerals and water left over after digestion and it stores the waste material. The stool is largely made up of byproducts of bacteria, and a small portion is nondigested things we eat. The large intestine pushes the stool down to the lower part of the intestine and into the rectum to be evacuated. This occurs automatically and at irregular intervals.

The ability to control bowel movements is related to tightening and relaxation of two circular muscles (sphincters) which circle the anus. The muscle near the outside of the anus is called the external sphincter, and comes under our voluntary control around two to three years of age. The circular muscle further inside, the internal sphincter, usually opens automatically when stool fills the rectum (the last part of the large bowel above the anus). Normally, we feel this happening and recognize the urge to have a bowel movement. We then keep the external sphincter closed until it is convenient to eliminate the waste, at which time the external sphincter is relaxed. Stool is pushed out by contraction of the rectum which is helped by tightening of the stomach muscles. The most effective position in which to have a bowel movement is the squatting position.

189

INTESTINAL SYSTEM

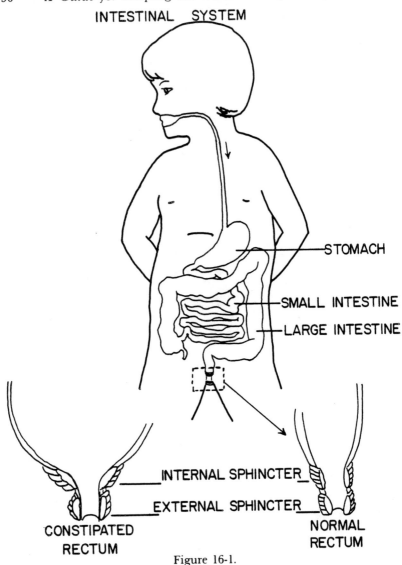

Figure 16-1.

Why Do Children with Spina Bifida Have Bowel Problems?

The nerves that supply the external sphincter come from the lowest level of the spinal cord. These lower nerves are damaged in nearly all children with spina bifida. Even children with no apparent abnormalities of the legs often do not have any control of the external anal sphincter. Also, depending on the level of the nerve damage, the child may or may not be able to feel the presence of stool in the rectum.

In children with spina bifida, the internal sphincter usually responds normally, i.e. when stool passes into the rectum, the internal anal sphincter relaxes. If the external anal sphincter is relaxed and the pressure of the propulsive contraction of the intestine, plus the pressure from the abdominal muscles is strong enough, stool will pass out through the anus. Since the child often does not feel the stool and cannot control the external sphincter, bowel control is difficult to achieve.

Usual Findings in the Child with Spina Bifida

(1) A normal involuntary internal anal sphincter response.
(2) Lack of control over the external anal sphincter.
(3) Absence of sensation when the rectum is full.
(4) Weak stomach muscles (used in pushing stool out).

Common Bowel Problems in the Child with Spina Bifida

As well as the incontinence and difficulty with toilet training mentioned above, children with spina bifida may have constipation, diarrhea, impaction, rectal prolapse, anal fissures, and skin problems around the anus. These problems will be discussed later.

Goals of a Bowel Training Program

The aim of a bowel training program is for regular emptying of the bowels with no leakage of stool in between. With careful management, these goals can be met in nearly all children with spina bifida. The training process is often lengthy and may have times of both encouragement and discouragement. The goal, however, is very gratifying to both child and parents when it is reached.

Developing Regular Toileting Habits

Bowel movements frequently follow eating. There is a stomach-large bowel ("gastro-colic") reflex in which stretching of the stomach causes reflex contractions of the colon. In toilet training, it helps if the parents take advantage of this reflex and place the child on the toilet shortly after meals. This also develops a regular time when bowel movements can conveniently occur, and this regularity is helpful in controlling when movements occur. The most effective position for a bowel movement is squatting, and the correct position on a comfortable toilet is important in teaching the child control.

Children with spina bifida have difficulty separating bladder and bowel control. If they have sufficient strength in stomach muscles to strain and empty the bladder, they will frequently empty the rectum at the same time. Laughing and crying may also empty the rectum of small amounts. Once a child learns to empty his bowel regularly, he is very close to controlling his bowel movements.

When Is a Child Ready to Begin Training?

Your child's readiness to be trained is somewhat individual. In general, he should start as soon as his friends begin, which is usually between two and three years of age. Be alert for the signs listed below. They are indications that you should be considering a bowel training program.

1. Does your child give any sign that he is about to have a bowel movement? Does he lie very quiet, strain or turn red in the face?
2. Can your child sit on a chair with a brace or support?
3. Is he able to sit on a potty seat for three to five minutes?
4. Is he aware of other family members using the toilet?
5. Is he familiar with words such as "potty, diaper, pants?"

Suggestions on Toilet Training

Toilet training can be attempted with a variety of approaches depending on your child's ability and personality. Generally a casual, good-humored and patient manner is most successful. Do not start toilet training when your child has diarrhea or sickness, or when the family is having some difficulties.

1. Choose a word for bowel movement that you will be using for bowel training and use it consistently when diapering.
2. Choose a potty chair with arms and be sure his feet will touch the floor or use a box to hold his legs and feet in position. His knees should be slightly higher than his buttocks to have advantage of gravity and to approximate a squatting position.
3. If possible, note the time of day when he usually has a bowel movement and place him on the potty for a short period near that time.
4. To begin with, place him on the potty at least once a day. This should be for approximately three to five minutes.
5. Verbally praise him anytime he is successful.
6. Teach him to push with his abdominal muscles so that he can do this while toileting. Blowing balloons or bubbles in water are useful exercises for this.
7. You may use gentle pressure on the abdomen (circular,

downward movement) especially on left side.

8. When he is on the toilet, finger pressure on the outside of the anus may help him to expel the stool.

9. Use of a mirror when the stool is coming or when the anus is opening may help him understand the desired results, since he may be unable to feel what is happening.

10. As his interest increases, the length of time he is placed on the toilet can be increased also. Start at three to five minutes, then gradually increase to 15 to 20 minutes as his tolerance allows. The frequency may also be increased to two to three times a day.

11. As he grows older, he may associate a feeling of mild cramping in the abdomen with the approach of a bowel movement. He should go quickly to the toilet.

12. Never show disappointment or displeasure if he cannot go.

Remember that bowel training takes time and patience, but children like to please their parents. Once it is accomplished, your child will be proud of his accomplishment and have a greater feeling of independence. He will also sense your pleasure and pride in his success. His success will also free some of your time for other pursuits, or perhaps just make your life a bit easier.

What If Toilet Training Is Difficult?

If you are having a great deal of difficulty in helping your child become toilet trained, an assisted evacuation program can be used. This should only be started with your doctor's supervision. You place him on the toilet seat or potty chair after breakfast or supper for about 15 minutes. If no bowel movement occurs spontaneously, then you insert one-half or one glycerin suppository. Allow the suppository 15 to 30 minutes to dissolve and take effect while the child is lying down. If necessary, the buttocks may be held together. Then you place him on the toilet seat or potty chair again. If no results are obtained within 60 minutes of inserting the suppository, you give a pediatric Fleet's® enema and after 15 to 30 minutes, again place him on the toilet. This daily program is usually followed for a two- to three-week period. With some children, it is quite effective in helping them evacuate daily in the toilet.

Why Does My Child Get Constipated?

Children with spina bifida often develop constipation when waste material accumulates in the large bowel. The large intestine automatically pushes waste through to the rectum, but movement of the stool out of the rectum is assisted by abdominal muscles. When these muscles are weak as in many children with spina bifida, they are not able to push as vigorously. If the stool is not passed out through the anus, it accumulates in the rectum. When stool remains in the rectum, it often becomes hard because more of its water content is absorbed back into the body. As the mass of stool increases, the rectum stretches. When this distention occurs over a long time, the rectum loses its ability to push the stool out. Therefore, a cycle of events is established, which, if not stopped, can mean long-term constipation. In general, constipation can often be avoided by a high roughage diet, adequate fluid intake and the development of good bowel habits.

Why Does My Child Get Diarrhea?

The causes of diarrhea in children with spina bifida are the same as for all children. They may develop an infection which irritates the bowel or they have diarrhea from a food intolerance. The most common food children become intolerant to is lactose, which is the sugar found in milk.

Since the external sphincter in children with spina bifida may not stay closed when stool is in the rectum, they may have constant soiling. This may be confused with diarrhea. Also, at times, a child may seem to have diarrhea when the problem is really an impaction. If your child has diarrhea frequently or for long periods, you should discuss it with your doctor.

Impaction

An impaction is the presence of a large collection of hard stool in the rectum. You may suspect it because of infrequent bowel movements, and your doctor can confirm it by feeling a mass of stool on an abdominal or rectal exam. You may be able to feel the lumps of stool in the lower abdomen by pressing gently in this area.

The child usually has frequent mushy stools in small amounts. When your doctor does a rectal exam, he will feel a hard mass of stool. This mass holds the sphincters open and, as a result, liquid stool slips around the mass and passes through. Since your child may not be able to contract the outside sphincter, he cannot prevent the stool from leaking.

If an impaction develops, it must be removed. This can be done by giving one or more enemas. Your doctor can help select which enema to use.

Using an Enema

Your doctor can help you with the solution to use. It might be warm salt water, tap water, or a ready-to-use disposable enema. A ready-to-use enema should be warmed by placing the closed container in warm water for a few minutes.

Place your child on his left side. Lubricate the tip of the enema tubing with Vaseline™ if it is not already lubricated. Allow a small amount of solution to run through the tubing and clamp it off. Insert the enema tip slowly and gently into your child's anus, going approximately two to three inches deep, depending on your child's size. Remember your child lacks sensation around the rectum and will generally not find this uncomfortable.

Release the clamp and let the solution flow in slowly to prevent cramping. In ready-to-use enemas, slowly roll the container so the solution is expelled. If leaking occurs around the tube, hold the buttocks together with your hand. Remove the tube and encourage your child to hold the solution as long as possilbe (15 to 30 minutes). He may need help holding it due to the weak muscles.

Place him on the toilet for the bowel movement. If the enema gives no results, you may have to put on a rubber glove and, with a lubricated finger, break up the hard mass. You should take care not to remove too large a piece at a time since you can injure the anus.

Enemas are occasionally used for completing evacuation, but the routine use of enemas for periodic evacuation is not recommended.

What Is a Rectal Prolapse?

Prolapse is the protrusion of the mucous lining of the rectum through the anus. This is caused by weak muscles and can occur when your child is passing bowel movements, has diarrhea, or is straining. You can gently replace the bowel with a lubricated gloved finger. If it occurs frequently, it may need to be surgically repaired. Your doctor can help decide. The repair is simple but requires hospitalization, since a stitch must be placed on the inside of the anus.

What Are Anal Fissures and Perianal Skin Problems?

Anal fissures are tears in the skin of the anus caused by the passage of large hard stools. They are treated by keeping the stool very soft for several months.

Frequent passage of loose stool may cause irritation of the skin around the anus. This may occur with diarrhea, impaction with soiling, or from continual dampness due to urine.

How To Prevent Constipation

With the regular emptying of the rectum, the problem of constipation, accidental passing of stool, impaction, and rectal prolapse may frequently be avoided. In some children, a high roughage diet with plenty of liquids will keep the bowel movements soft enough to pass easily so they can regularly empty the rectum. Unabsorbable fiber in the diet helps retain water in the bowel to keep the stool soft and easily passed.

Fluid (six to eight glasses per day), *fiber* (hull, bran, vegetable and fruit skin and other hard to digest parts of food) and certain *laxative foods* (yeast, prunes, bran) in the child's diet will help reduce any tendency towards constipation. Certain foods such as milk and cheese, tend to be constipating, and should be limited in quantity. Appendix F outlines other mealtime suggestions to assist in bowel control.

Often a child will follow his parent's example about likes and dislikes, so you should also try to eat a well-balanced, high-fiber diet. Food should be attractively served and in small enough portions so as not to discourage the young child with a small appetite. Appetites are variable and will change with the age of the child. Starting bran early in life will accustom him to the taste. Insist on a taste of the new food when he is hungry and not when he is full.

The atmosphere at the dinner table may determine how well your child will eat. Mealtime should be a happy time for the whole family. Try to avoid undue stress, punishment, constant correction of faulty manners, and long dinners for small children. Good conversation helps.

Studies have been done with children which show that they are more apt to eat what they help to prepare. Having them peel carrots, mix cookie batter, and make hamburger patties may help.

Your child needs every opportunity to show his independence. This will help his bowel program over the long run as well as his overall development and feeling of self-importance.

What Role Do Medications Play?

Dietary management is the most important, but laxatives may be used as an aid to improve bowel function *while* the appetite and habit are being appropriately trained. It is important to check with your doctor about the right medication and dose for your child's size and his bowel pattern.

There are four different types of laxatives. They are the intestinal muscle stimulants, the osmotic laxatives, bulk-forming laxatives, and the softening laxatives.

Laxatives that Stimulate the Intestinal Muscles

These produce results by making the intestine contract and try to empty itself. These medications increase the muscle tone of the large intestine. In high doses, they produce cramps, especially if the stools are hard.

Specific examples of such laxatives include the following: castor oil — very strong, works in one to two hours; phenophthalein (Ex-Lax®, Feen-A-Mint® and others), mild, works in six to eight hours and the effect may last for a day or two, not safe for long-term use; senna (Senokot®), mild, works in six to twelve hours, available as liquid, granules, and tablets; Dulcolax® — available in suppositories as well as pills, mild, works in six to twelve hours orally, 10 to 30 minutes rectally; cascara, castoria, etc. — mild, works in about eight hours.

Osmotic Laxatives

These produce soft stools by drawing water out of the body and into the stool. They contain magnesium and can be harmful if kidney disease is present. They are seldom used in children with spina bifida. They are relatively mild and work in six to twelve hours. Examples include: milk of magnesia, epsom salts, magnesium carbonate, magnesium citrate, and sodium phosphate.

Bulk-forming Laxatives

These agents produce soft stools by retaining water in the stool. They are the least irritating to the body and quite effective if the dose is adequate. They begin to work in one to two days. There is very little direct stimulating effect on the intestinal muscle. Examples include: bran (cereals, bread, bran muffins, etc.), psyllium (Konsyl®, Metamucil®, LA Formula®), methylcellulose, and agar.

Stool-softening Laxatives

These agents work directly to make the stool soft. They do not stimulate evacuation. They are effective in one to three days. Examples include: Colace®, Doxinate®,. Surfak®, mineral oil.

Laxatives such as Colace, Doxinate, Surfak, Magcyl®, and Polykol® are wetting agents and make the stool mass water soluble. They can soften a hard stool which is present in the rectum. They should not be used with mineral oil, because they enable the mineral oil to be absorbed by the intestine.

Mineral oil keeps the stools from getting hard and lubricates the stool that is already formed. It minimally interferes with the absorption of fat soluble vitamins A and D. A variety of flavored mineral oil preparations or combinations are available on the market. Examples are Petrogalar®, Agoral®, Kondremul®, and Zymenol®.

Rectal Suppositories

Rectal suppositories are small lumps of medication which are inserted into the rectum through the anus. They are often used with a bowel training program. A suppository may be given once a day to help the child have a good bowel movement at a regular time. Examples include: glycerin, an osmotic laxative, very gentle, works in 30 to 60 minutes; Dulcolax, a stimulant laxative, very effective works in 15 to 60 mintues.

Uses and Side Effects of Medications

A daily dose of an osmotic or a stimulant laxative is often used to keep the rectum cleaned out. If evacuation occurs daily, but the stools are hard, the bulk forming agents or the softening agents are useful. Too much of a stimulant laxative can produce abdominal cramps or diarrhea. The chronic use of stimulant laxatives over many years may lead to a colon which does not respond to these medications. Giving too much mineral oil may result in the oil leaking out through the rectum.

Some children may need these medications regularly over a long time interval while their bowel habits are being established. Your physician can help you choose the appropriate medication and the amount so that the common side effects can be avoided. A well-guided medication program can assist your child in learning to control his bowels, and eventually the medication can be decreased. If you find he needs increasing amounts of medication to control his bowel movements, your physician should reevaluate his program.

CHAPTER 17

THE URINARY SYSTEM

THE urinary system is a vital part of the functioning of every human body. It consists of the kidneys, which produce the urine, and a system of tubes which carry the urine out of the body. This urinary system is closely related to the genital system which is important in sexual functioning. Both systems are usually considered together and termed the genitourinary system. The kidneys are the key part of the urinary system. They remove excess water and waste materials from the body and assist in regulating the chemicals in the blood. These functions are needed for life itself; and when the kidneys can no longer provide this service, death occurs.

Children with spina bifida nearly all have a urinary system which does not function properly. Fortunately, the kidneys are usually normal, and the damage is only to the parts of the system which control how the body eliminates urine. In other words, children with spina bifida usually begin life with the most important part of the system (the kidneys) working normally. Unfortunately, the parts which do not work properly can eventually lead to kidney damage unless proper care is provided.

The urinary problems experienced by children with spina bifida are very similar to those present in patients who have injuries to the spinal cord. Spinal cord damage is frequently seen in injured soldiers and victims of auto accidents, and many centers around the world have developed methods of handling the resulting problems. These advances have been modified and are now used to help children with spina bifida.

In developing a plan to care for the genitourinary system in the child with spina bifida, there are certain priorities which should be followed. The goal is to save or improve the three basic functions; that is, the kidney function, bladder function, and sexual function. Kidney function is basic to life itself, while bladder function is basic to social acceptance; and sexual function is basic to self-esteem.

How the Kidneys and Urinary System Work

We are all born with approximately five times as much kidney tissue as we need to provide what is considered normal kidney function. There are generally two kidneys, and each one contains millions of tiny filters which help regulate many processes in the body. These

199

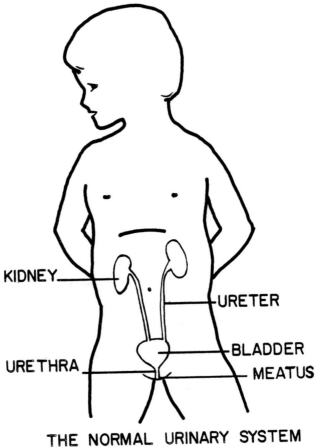

THE NORMAL URINARY SYSTEM

Figure 17-1.

filters and other parts of the kidney help control the excretion of water, the maintenance of an acid and salt balance in the blood, the regulation of blood pressure, and the production of blood cells. Saving the kidney so it can perform these functions is one of the most important goals of health care.

From each kidney, there is a small tube, the ureter, through which urine drains into the bladder. Each ureter enters the bladder at an angle and, thus, forms a flap valve which prevents urine from flowing backwards from the bladder back up into the kidney. When this flap valve does not work, there is a reflux or a return of urine from the bladder back to the kidney. If this urine is infected, it can cause infection and serious damage to the kidney.

From the bladder, urine passes through a channel, the urethra, to the outside. The urethra is surrounded by a muscle which can open or close this channel. The muscle is circular with the channel through the middle and is called the urinary sphincter. When the sphincter is closed, urine cannot leave the bladder. The sphincter and bladder work together in controlling how urine is eliminated. The bladder is a muscular sac which stores the urine. It can hold about a cup of urine at birth and up to three pints in the adult. Periodically, the bladder

THE DIFFERENCE BETWEEN THE MALE AND FEMALE URINARY SYSTEM. NOTICE THE LONGER DISTANCE FROM THE OUTSIDE TO THE BLADDER IN THE MALE.

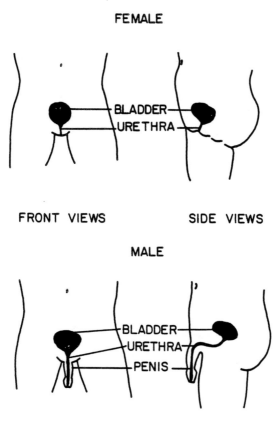

Figure 17-2.

tightens, and if the sphincter relaxes and opens then urine is passed. If the sphincter is closed, then urine cannot pass through the urethra, and the bladder relaxes again. When the bladder contracts and urine does pass, the bladder automatically empties all of the urine present.

The normal control of urination is complicated, and some details of how it functions are unknown. Several parts of the brain, the spinal cord, and nerves to the genitourinary system are intimately involved in coordinating urination. Because there are so many nerve pathways and interconnections involved in the control of urination, most children with spina bifida have urinary problems.

Why Does Spina Bifida Cause Urine Problems?

There are many ways that damage to the nervous system can affect the bladder in children with spina bifida. Whenever the bladder does not work correctly, because its nervous connections are not right, the term neurogenic bladder is used. Usually the bladder, kidneys and connecting tubes are normal in the beginning, but the loss of nervous control over them leads to changes. There are two major ways that nervous system damage affects the bladder. One makes the bladder muscle very relaxed (flaccid bladder), while the other makes it irritable and tight (spastic bladder).

When the bladder muscle is limp or relaxed (flaccid bladder), it is unable to tighten completely and force all of the urine out. Therefore, when the bladder fills, it may remain full. Any more urine that enters will simply dribble out through the urethra. This urine leakage can occur continually. In addition, when pressure is put on the bladder, such as by pushing on the abdomen, laughing, crying, or straining, even more urine leaks out. Despite this leaking of urine and the bladder tightening partially, there is always urine remaining. This is termed residual urine.

When the bladder muscle is irritable and tight (spastic bladder), then it does not act as a storage place for urine. Whenever a small amount of urine enters the bladder, the muscle tightens and urine leaks out. Again, the bladder does not completely empty, so some urine usually remains.

Pressure develops within the bladder when it contracts. This pressure forces urine out of the bladder. There are two tubes that bring urine from the kidneys to the bladder (ureters) and one that takes urine to the outside of the body (urethra). Pressure within the bladder usually forces the urine to the outside of the body through the urethra. When the system is not working correctly, however, the pressure can sometimes force the urine back up into the kidneys. This causes the drainage system (ureters) from the kidneys to enlarge, a condition called hydronephrosis.

Urine which remains in the bladder or ureters presents a problem,

THREE TYPES OF BLADDERS

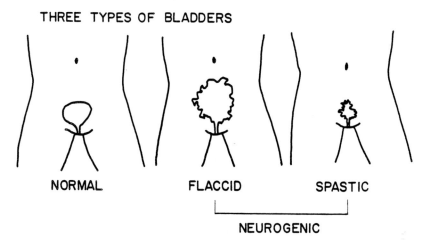

NORMAL   FLACCID   SPASTIC

NEUROGENIC

Figure 17-3.

because it provides a place for bacteria to grow. The urine can become infected very easily. This is especially true in girls, since the distance from the skin to bladder is shorter than in boys. Consequently, bacteria from the skin can reach the bladder more easily. If infected urine backs up into the ureters, a kidney infection can result. Both the pressure from backed up urine and the presence of infection can lead to kidney damage if they persist for many months.

The goals in treating the urinary system are to help the urine drain completely in a way which the child can partially or completely control and to prevent urine infection.

How to Help Prevent Infection

There are several ways you can reduce the chances that the urine will become infected. A large fluid intake is helpful since it flushes out the bladder frequently. Thus, bacteria do not have much time to grow.

An acid urine also helps, since bacteria grow poorly if the urine is acid. Vitamin C, fruit juices, and medications such as Mandelamine® and naladixic acid all help make the urine acid and decrease infection.

It is important to completely empty the bladder of urine in order to prevent the growth of bacteria. For some children, firm pressure on the lower abdomen (called Credé's method) will force the bladder to empty. As the child grows older, he can do this himself by using his hand or by tightening his stomach muscles. This Credé's method or maneuver pushes on the bladder and helps expel the residual urine. This should be done every three or four hours. However, since pressure on the bladder occasionally causes urine to flow back up to the kidneys, you should check with your physician before using Credé's method.

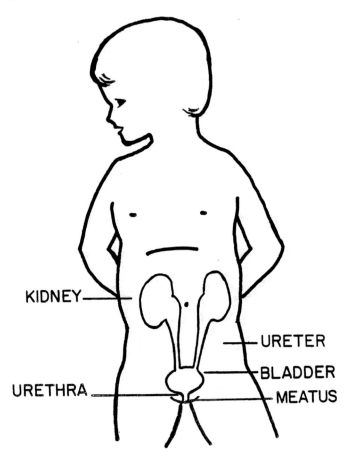

REFLUX AND HYDRONEPHROSIS

Figure 17-4.

How Can You Tell If the Urine Is Infected?

Discomfort and frequent urination are common signs of urine infection, but children with spina bifida have little or no feeling around the bladder and genitalia. Therefore, they may not feel burning when they urinate, have bladder pain, or recognize an increased need to urinate. More commonly in children with spina bifida, a strong odor or cloudy urine is an early sign of infection. Fever or vomiting without other cause may also be due to urine infection. Other children have stomach pain or develop skin sores from the infected urine. If the kidneys are infected, there may also be back pain.

How Can Your Doctor Recognize the Infection?

By looking at the urine under a microscope, your doctor can see evidence of infection. However, the final answer comes from culturing the urine and growing the bacteria. A culture of the urine takes at least one to two days. The culture and testing the bacteria for their sensitivity to various antibiotics is the best way for your doctor to determine which medication will be most effective for this infection. Since children with spina bifida may have frequent urine infections, the most effective antibiotic may change. Culture and sensitivity tests are necessary to recognize this change.

What If the Urine Is Infected?

If the doctor finds a urine infection, he will begin your child on antibiotics. If your child continues to have infections after the treatment, your doctor may keep him on a small dose of antibiotic each day in an effort to prevent further infections. It is important to have follow-up urine cultures to be sure the antibiotic is effective in controlling infection. The child with repeated urine infections may also benefit from better bladder drainage using intermittent catheterization. This method is discussed in detail in the next chapter.

Tests Used to Examine Kidney Function

BLOOD TESTS. By measuring chemicals that the kidney removes from the blood, your doctor can tell how well the kidneys are doing their job. Creatinine and BUN (blood urea nitrogen) are two such tests.

URINE TESTS. In addition to examining and culturing the urine, there is a test of the kidney filtering ability which can be done. This is called a Creatinine Clearance, and it requires both a blood sample and a 24-hour urine sample.

X-RAYS. An intravenous pyelogram IVP is an x-ray study which is an excellent method for evaluating the urinary tract. A dye is injected into a vein. When the kidneys function properly, this dye is excreted through the tiny kidney filters and drains into the bladder. The dye outlines the kidneys on x-rays and shows the kidney structure. If the kidneys, ureters or bladder are dilated from backed up urine, this can be seen. Areas of the kidney that are damaged, scarred or dilated can also be seen.

Tests Used to Check the Bladder

X-RAYS. A more specific x-ray of the bladder is the voiding cystoure-throgram (VCUG). In this test, a catheter is passed into the bladder through the urethra. The bladder is then filled with dye and x-rays are taken to see the outline of the bladder. The catheter is then removed and x-rays are again taken while the child passes urine. If the dye in the bladder backs up into the kidneys (reflux), this can be seen. This x-ray also shows how completely the child empties the bladder. If the bladder does not empty completely, then dye will be present in it after the child passes urine.

CYSTOSCOPY. This is a procedure that allows the doctor to look inside the bladder through a large catheter. Usually, children are put to sleep for cystoscopy. This procedure may be combined with other measurements.

THE CYSTOMETROGRAM. The pressure in the bladder at various volumes is measured by this instrument. The child is catheterized and the bladder filled with fluid or gas. The pressure in the bladder is measured as the amount of fluid or gas increases. If the bladder muscle is overactive (spastic) or not active (flaccid), it will be seen on this test.

THE URETHRAL PRESSURE PROFILE. A catheter is slowly withdrawn from the bladder and the pressure is measured at each point along the urethra. By comparing the pressure in the bladder and the pressure in the urethra, the pressure where urine leakage will occur can be predicted.

OTHER TESTS. More sophisticated tests of the nerve supply to the bladder and pressures within the bladder and urethra are called urodynamics. This is a group of tests which can provide accurate information about the bladder and urethra. They are not done routinely, but only when there is a special indication. There are two main functions of the bladder: storing and emptying urine. The bladder stores urine as long as its pressure is less than that in the urethra and sphincter muscles. Urodynamics measures these pressures. Therefore, these pressures are valuable in determining how the urinary tract is functioning.

How to Have Good Bladder Function

Once damage to the nerves has occurred, such as with spina bifida, the goal is to seek the best possible balance between the two bladder functions of urine storage and emptying. The ideal goal is to have enough urine storage to prevent or lessen urinary leakage and enough emptying so that very little urine remains in the bladder after voiding (residual urine). There are a number of maneuvers that can be used to achieve these ends, and commonly more than one is required. The simplest method of therapy should be tried first.

If the main problem is that of storing urine, then there are two ways to proceed. A number of medications are available which relax the bladder and increase the bladder capacity, so it can hold urine for a longer period of time. Other medicines tighten the sphincter muscle and further help to store urine. Also, surgery is sometimes used to tighten the urethra.

When the main problem is emptying the bladder, then it is essential to decrease the pressure in the urethra or increase the pressure in the bladder. Again, various medications alone, or in combination, can assist in achieving this. The Credé's maneuver mentioned earlier is another way to help empty the bladder.

At present, clean intermittent self-catheterization for both boys and girls is probably the most effective, least costly, and safest way to empty the bladder. It has a number of advantages and enables the bladder to be completely emptied at intervals. Combining this procedure with medications to stop the bladder from contracting helps to maintain dryness. Completely emptying the bladder also helps control infection. This technique is discussed in more detail in the next chapter.

When Should Urine Be Diverted from the Bladder?

In spite of medications, various operations, Credé's maneuver, and intermittent catheterization, a few children with spina bifida will still require a permanent urinary diversion. These are generally children who have problems with bladder storage and emptying and also have significant damage to their kidneys. In the past, an ileal loop or conduit was the preferred technique. This operation consists of disconnecting the ureters from the bladder and a piece of small intestine (ileum) from the rest of the gastrointestinal tract. Next, the ureters are stitched to the ileum and the ileum stiched to the abdominal wall to form an opening or stoma. Urine drains continuously through the ileum and out the stoma. Long-term studies of children who have undergone this operation reveal some problems. One problem is that the surgeon cannot construct a flap valve where the ureter enters the ileum. Thus, urine can flow freely backwards up to the kidneys. This can transmit infection, as well as pressure, to the kidneys. More recently, this problem has been lessened by using a different part of the intestine, so that a flap valve can be constructed and reflux prevented. With this new technique, there are also fewer problems with the stoma.

Future Possibilities for Bladder Control

Ideally, it would be best if a device to control urination could be hidden internally and there would be no need for medicines, a stoma, or a catheter. Electrical stimulators to make the bladder contract have been tried, but are not very successful. These devices stimulate the bladder to contract by applying an electrical current, but the amount of current required is so great that nerves elsewhere are also stimulated and cause various side effects.

Another ingenious method has been devised. This method involves surgically placing an inflatable cuff around the urethra. The cuff can then be inflated to prevent urination and deflated when the patient wishes to void. For this method to work, any nerve control the individual may have over urination must be surgically removed. If a complication should occur and the child be unable to use the device, irreversible changes have already been made. When a mechanical device is used to control urination, a regular pattern of urinating must be followed or serious problems can result.

Both types of devices are made of materials not normally found in the body. These foreign bodies can become infected, and like any mechanical device, they can malfunction. Active investigation is currently underway to improve present techniques for handling these urine problems.

TAKING CARE OF WET PANTS

Achieving dry pants is one of the greatest steps your child can take in gaining control over his body. A sense of self-control will foster good feelings about his body (body image) and good overall feelings about himself (self-esteem). Your child's further accomplishments in independence and care of himself depends on this initial achievement.

Failure to achieve dry pants at the same age as friends has a serious negative effect on children. In the language of children, they "feel like a baby" when they have to wear diapers beyond the normal length of time. This is your child's way of acknowledging a lack of control over his body and expressing negative feelings about himself.

Our society accepts children in wet pants until around the age of three. At that point, adults and children alike notice the presence of diapers. For the parents of an incontinent child, these can be trying times. You may have to contend with implications from uninformed individuals that you are neglecting your duties because your child is not toilet-trained. You may wonder yourself about the source of your child's incontinence, even though you understand about nerve damage from spina bifida. It is sometimes hard to escape the feeling that your child is wetting because he is lazy. A brief explanation of the reason for your child's wetting may help you deal with friends and establish realistic expectations for your child.

Your child is not receiving signals from his body that it is time to urinate, as is the average child. The same generally holds true for bowel movements. Some children receive more signals than others; but it is safe to say that young children with spina bifida have a hard

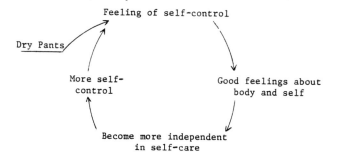

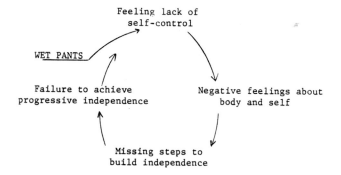

Success encourages more success

Feeling of self-control

Dry Pants

More self-control

Good feelings about body and self

Become more independent in self-care

Progress is based on prior accomplishments

6 Experience more self-control

5 Become more independent in self-care

4 Good feelings about entire self

3 Good feelings about body

2 Feeling of self-control

Step #1 Dry pants

Lack of success discourages future success

Feeling lack of self-control

WET PANTS

Failure to achieve progressive independence

Negative feelings about body and self

Missing steps to build independence

Progress cannot occur without prior accomplishments

Step # 1 Wet pants

2 Feeling of lack of self-control

3 Negative feelings about body

4 Negative feelings about entire self

5 Missing steps to build independence

6 Failure to achieve progressive independence

time decoding the signals they receive, if any. This makes achieving dry pants especially challenging. However, something can be done about the problem.

Bathroom Routine

A program for taking care of wet pants is designed to compensate for what your child lacks due to nerve damage from the spina bifida. A bathroom routine can partly compensate for the absence of the usual sensation. A bathroom routine simply means that your child goes to the toilet on a regular schedule. An example of a reasonable toilet schedule is the following:

7 AM	10 AM	12 noon	2:30 PM	5:30 PM	8:30 PM
arising	mid-morning	lunchtime	before school	after	before bed
	at school	at school	bus arrives	supper	

Since children with spina bifida often dribble urine, a schedule of regular toileting by itself may not guarantee complete dryness. It is, however, the first logical step toward becoming dry. It is also the foundation of eventual bowel control.

A regular bathroom routine will have the following important results:

(1) Familiarizes your child with the appropriate time for urination and defecation and introduces the beginnings of discipline.

(2) Gets your child used to the bathroom and sitting on a potty so that it is not a fearsome event.

(3) Offers you an opportunity to positively reinforce your child for trying.

(4) Contributes to your child's sense of active participation in controlling his body function.

(5) Lays the foundation for your child accepting personal responsibility for a function that other children normally handle.

Useful Equipment

DIAPERS. It is likely that your child will be wearing diapers longer than average. Most parents prefer disposable diapers. With some stretching, these fit until the age of about five years. The major companies have not found it financially profitable to produce larger diapers, because there is such a small demand. However, there are manufacturers of large disposable diapers. They primarily supply institutions such as hospitals and nursing homes. Occasionally, they will sell to private consumers, but usually only in large quantities. Purchasing large diapers in bulk could be feasible if several parents cooperated and then divided them.

INCONTINENCE PANTS. Around the time your child is becoming too large for diapers, another more sophisticated choice becomes available. Several companies now are producing incontinence pants in children's sizes. These pants are a cross between a diaper and underwear and will probably represent to your child a graduation from baby-like diapers.* The pants are fairly successful and generally more acceptable to children than the rubber pants which balloon under trousers and dresses.

Whatever style incontinence pants you choose, they are fitted pri-

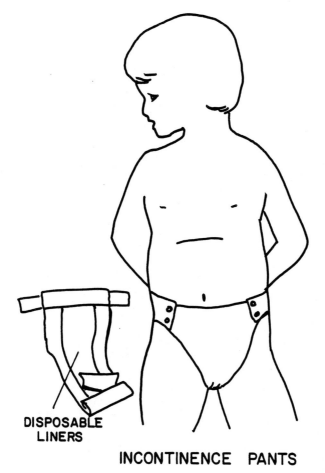

DISPOSABLE LINERS

INCONTINENCE PANTS

Figure 17-5.

---

marily to waist size and designed for small adults. Consequently, the leg holes are often too large. The market for children's size incontinence pants is a recent one in the United States, and garment producers might welcome suggestions from parents on how to better construct their product.

URINE COLLECTING DEVICES. Boys have another choice which is made possible by their anatomy. They can be fitted with an external device which fits over the penis. It collects the urine and drains it into a bag which is usually strapped to the leg. This leg bag must be emptied on a regular schedule, depending on your child's size, the volume of the bag, and his fluid intake. A children's market for these

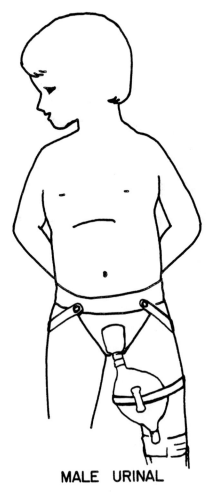

MALE URINAL

Figure 17-6.

devices is again recent, and manufacturers are just beginning to design products for children's needs. With suggestions from parents, they could perhaps create better appliances than exist today.

The urine collecting appliances can be fitted to boys as young as four years. They are ordered by waist and penis size. You may have to make a few adjustments at home to ensure a personalized fit for your child. Local surgical supply stores may carry a stock or they can order a special appliance for you.

For some boys a penile appliance represents a great improvement over diapers or incontinence pants. They must take some responsibility in emptying the bag and learn how to manage their equipment. For some children this provides a sense of achievement, but others are bothered by the artificial nature of the appliance. Associated problems, such as difficulty fitting boys who have a small penis and spillage when an active boy twists or parts of the equipment come unstuck, also bother some children. Equipment must be kept meticulously clean or it may have an odor.

There are other appliances which stick directly onto the penis, but they are generally not effective for children. Despite improved sticking products, it is difficult to keep a condom in place over the penis of an active child. Additionally, small boys generally have a small penis which makes it difficult to attach a condom. Condom-type devices also have a tendency to twist and block the urine from the condom down to the leg bag. This can result in urine backing up and spilling onto clothes. Manufacturers have attempted to prevent this by placing a plastic cup in the condom. This has reduced the twisting problem, but creates an area where urine tends to pool and keep the penis wet.

Poor drainage into the leg bag may be a problem at nap time if the child's position prevents gravity from draining the urine. Nighttime drainage sets are available for drainage when the child is in a lying position. However, it is not a good idea to use a urine collecting appliance 24 hours a day. Skin needs to be exposed to air and nighttime is usually the most convenient time to do this. If the penis remains constantly moist, ulcerations can develop from contact with ammonia in the urine.

There are many effective products on the market and a device that is successful on one child may not be so on another. Some of this equipment is costly since manufacturers include the cost of development and distribution to a relatively small market.

Medications to Help with Incontinence

There are certain medications that may help your child achieve staying dry. Most medications work by increasing the bladder's capacity to accumulate urine so that a larger amount can be passed at one time, rather than small amounts dribbling constantly. These medications work in a variety of ways and need to be carefully selected by your child's physician, based upon the unique characteristics of your child and his bladder.

Some children are able to stay dry for longer periods with medications, but others are not benefited. Those children who do improve with medication continue to need a regular bathroom routine. Although the periods of being dry can be prolonged with a combination of medications and a bathroom routine, it is unusual for complete dryness to be achieved by these methods alone.

Children with spina bifida generally require larger doses of these medications than other children with similar problems, and parents need to be aware of possible medication side effects. Finding the most effective dosage of any medication, or the best combinations of medication, may take considerable time. Should side effects occur, they can usually be eliminated by changing the dosage or substituting one medication for another. These medications can be used in young children for the proper indications. Their effectiveness usually outweighs the risk of any side effects.

The common side effects of the frequently used drugs are as follows:

Tofranil® — Sleep disturbances, irritability, dry mouth, skin rash, ringing ears, tingly palms, nausea and vomiting.

Ditropan® — Dry mouth, blurred vision, dizziness, vomiting, skin rashes.

Ephedrine Sulfate — Rapid heart rate, increased blood pressure, insomnia.

Clean Intermittent Self-catheterization

The methods of managing wet pants described thus far are all helpful to some degree. However, they do not deal as directly with the source of the wetting as does the program called *clean intermittent self-catherization*. This program is thus rapidly becoming the treatment of choice for many children and is replacing other methods of managing wetness and urinary tract infection.

This program teaches children to place a clean catheter into their bladder every three to four hours. The purpose is to periodically completely drain the bladder of urine. This usually prolongs the child's periods of dryness and reduces the number of urinary tract infections. Total dryness and freedom from infection are not guaranteed on this program, but for many children the results are a great improvement over other approaches.

There are several principles which underlie this program. The major ones are as follows:

(1) The source of most wetting is incomplete emptying of the bladder.

(2) Periodically, children with a neurogenic bladder need to empty

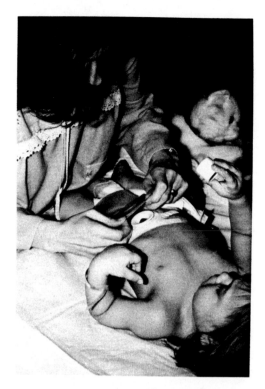

Putting on a Ileostomy Bag.

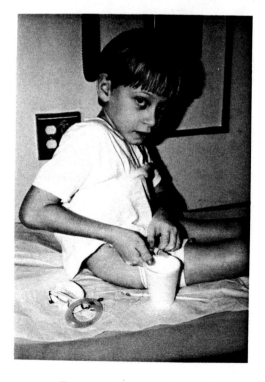

Emptying Ileostomy Bag.

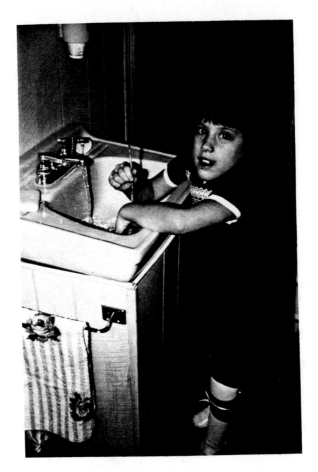

Washing Catheter.

their bladder completely.

(3) A neurogenic bladder needs special treatment.

(4) One cause of repeated urinary tract infections is a bladder which always contains too much urine. The presence of too much urine causes pressure against the bladder wall and slows the blood supply. This can decrease the bladder's ability to resist infection.

(5) Infected urine does not usually result from germs introduced by the catheter, if the bladder is regularly emptied completely.

The effectiveness of self-catheterization can sometimes be improved by medications. Such medications as Tofranil, Ditropan and Ephedrine, in combination with catheterization, can help some children achieve regular three to four hour periods of dryness during the day. This places the child with spina bifida roughly on a par with the general population; who also have to stop at the bathroom every three to four hours.

Some children are not candidates for the catheterization program. They are often boys who cannot tolerate the passage of the catheter or children who have the type of neurogenic bladder which does not store urine well. Other children cannot use their hands adequately, lack the mental ability, are emotionally too immature, or have families who feel unable to invest the required time.

Occasionally, children will need to stay on long-term antibiotics when on this program. These are usually children who have an accompanying urologic problem or who have been infected while on clean intermittent self-catheterization.

When Is My Child Ready to Catheterize Himself?

There do seem to be differences between boys and girls in determining readiness. Generally, boys can begin earlier than girls because they can visualize the target more easily. Overall degree of disability seems to be another factor. The less disabled a child, the earlier he can begin. There are some boys who are catheterizing themselves at four and others who have difficulty even when they are teenagers. The average age for both boys and girls would be around six to seven years. However, each child needs to be assessed individually and there are many factors to take into consideration. Some of these are the following:

1. The child's age.
2. The family's willingness to devote time to the project.
3. The interest and motivation of the child.
4. The child's ability to understand what he has to do and why.
5. The child's dexterity. The child's physical, mental and emotional abilities.
6. The ability to get his pants up and down as well as manipulate

braces and other equipment.
7. The ability to transfer onto the toilet.
8. The beginning of some regularity with bowel movements so that urinary control matches bowel control.

Although it would be desirable for all of these factors to be present before beginning, this is not necessary. Items one through five are the most important, but items six to eight should be at least in the developing stages. The prospect of starting a catheterization program may serve as an inspiration for some children to work harder on accomplishing these items.

Parents Catheterizing Their Children

The program of Clean Intermittent Self-Catheterization represents one of the best opportunities for a child to demonstrate control over his own bodily functions. For that reason, it is ideal if your child performs the catheterization himself, and leaves only what is absolutely necessary to an adult. Occasionally, children who have repeated urinary tract infections benefit from routine emptying of the bladder. If the child is very young, a parent can be taught this technique. However, it is generally best to wait until your child is old enough to start the program himself, unless there are medical reasons for starting earlier. This will avoid a potentially difficult transition period when responsibility is transferred from parent to child.

Teaching Children to Catheterize

Usually this technique is taught by a nurse who is familiar with spina bifida. This helps make the teaching a special event, and also relieves the parents of some responsibility for starting the program.
A usual teaching session would involve:
1. Explaining the rules of the program.
   A. hand washing
   B. lubricating the catheter (for boys)
   C. catheter washing and storage
   D. the schedule for catheterization
2. Viewing the anatomy on a diagram and discussing what catheterization does
3. Viewing their own anatomies
4. Touching their own anatomies
5. Finding the best position to catheterize themselves
6. Watching someone catheterize them
7. Helping catheterize themselves
8. Trying to catheterize themselves
9. Practicing catheterization

Parents are generally in the background for support, but are not encouraged to take a major part in the program. After they return home, the parent may need to remind a child when it is time to catheterize himself, or initially even help him find the right spot for the catheter. With encouragement and an opportunity to practice, catheterization becomes second nature in time.

Since a part of each child's day is usually spent in school, it is important that the school nurse be involved in the program. The nurse can be most helpful as a child is just beginning to learn. She can also help arrange the best time and place for catheterization so the child will have privacy and the school day will not be too disrupted.

Catheterization will need to be performed approximately every three to four hours during the day, unless a different timing is selected by your urologist and nurse. Catheterizing more frequently is quite demanding on children, and usually not needed. Catheterizing less frequently may result in spilling over of urine from a bladder which is too full. It is well to catheterize the bladder on arising in the morning since it is usually very full. Catheterizing before bed helps to minimize the urine that is in the bladder during the night and consequently decreases wetting. Children need their sleep and catheterizing at night is not necessary. Daytime dryness is the first priority for social reasons, and sometimes nighttime dryness occurs simply by virtue of a regular emptying program during the day.

Once the program starts, it is important to be faithful because the regular emptying (as opposed to irregular emptying) may influence the therapeutic effect. Regular emptying is so important that catheterization should occur even though water and soap for washing hands is not available. There will not, however, be any ill effects if circumstances occasionally prevent catheterization from occurring at the designated time.

The child will need regular health care visits while on the self-catheterization program. Routine urine samples should be taken during the early months of the program since urinary tract infections can occur. Medications to prolong the periods of dryness may be helpful, depending on the results obtained with catheterization alone.

THE ILEAL CONDUIT

Ileal conduits are primarily used to prevent progressive kidney disease. Only a few of the children with spina bifida develop the serious kidney changes which require this operation or a similar one in an effort to halt the progressive damage. The operation changes the flow of urine from the kidney so it bypasses the bladder. This eliminates some of the problems associated with a bladder that does not function properly. In the past, this surgery was also used to help children become dry; but with the development of other methods, this is no longer necessary.

What to Expect Before Surgery

Your child needs to be appropriately prepared for this type of surgery (see Hospitalization). To help prepare him, you should know what will happen before and after the surgery.

Some hospitals employ a specialist in the care of artificial openings such as ileal conduits. This individual is termed an enterostomal therapist, and is skilled in handling stomas or artificial openings on the body. They can also provide emotional support during and after this procedure.

The placement on the abdomen for the opening (or stoma) from which the urine will flow is one of the first decisions made. The position will depend on your child's activities, size, and past scars. Your child will need to be able to visualize the stoma easily so he can care for himself. The proposed opening is marked on the abdomen prior to surgery, and the urine collecting equipment tested before the operation. The child can then get the "feel" of the collecting equipment and any skin reactions to the materials can be detected. This will help him feel more comfortable about the operation and allow selection of the best equipment before it is actually needed.

Following surgery, he will return from the recovery room with the collecting equipment in place. The urine collecting equipment consists of a bag which fits over the stoma, and a long tube from the bag to the bedside collector. This system allows urine to drain away from the stoma while healing takes place and prevent any pull on the stoma from a heavy bag full of urine. When healing is complete, the tubing for constant drainage will not be needed during the daytime. Instead, a simple bag or appliance which fits over the stoma will be used. This bag needs to be emptied periodically, and will require a bathroom routine.

Immediately after the operation, the stoma may appear very large. The stoma, but not the connections inside, generally gets smaller with time. There will also be two small tubes emerging from the center of the stoma. They keep the inner portion of the operated area dry at the point where the ureters are connected to the piece of intestine or conduit. They will be removed in a few days. When they are removed, it is time to fit the appliance that your child will use after discharge.

What Type of Equipment Should Be Purchased?

The choice of equipment should be made with the help of a trained or experienced person. Over forty companies make products for ileal conduits. Therefore, you need help from someone with experience to know what is on the market, the merits of each product, and what is

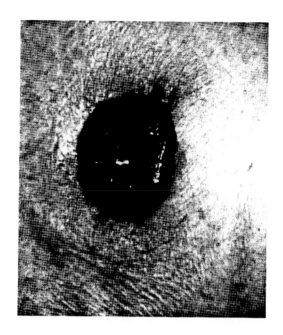

Plate I-1.
Normal stoma.

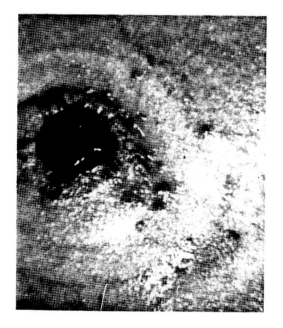

Plate I-2.
Skin irritation.

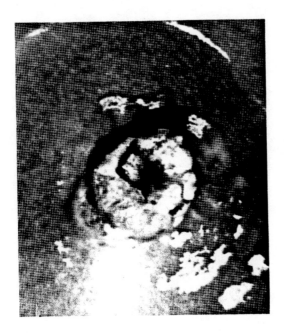

Plate II-1.
Alkaline urine.

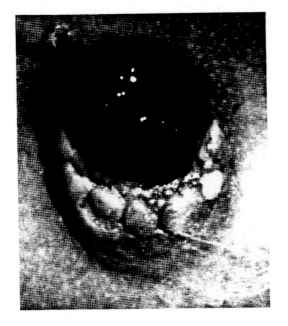

Plate II-2.
Alkaline urine and pseudo-epitheliomatous hyperplasia.

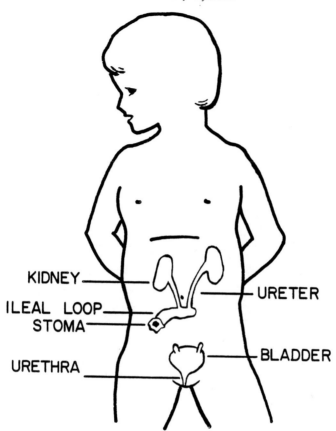

**THE URINARY SYSTEM
AFTER AN ILEAL LOOP**

Figure 17-7.

best for an individual child.

Equipment must suit both your child's *body* (overall size, oil content of skin, folds of fat, curves which occur due to position or anatomy) and his daily activities (brace walking, sitting in wheelchair, crawling, lying in bed, swimming). Ileal conduit equipment needs to be custom selected and should reflect the individuality of the child who wears it.

Since the size and shape of the stoma is expected to change after surgery, the stoma should be checked and the equipment reevaluated frequently during the first year. If there are any questions regarding the fit of the appliance, they should be dealt with when they arise. It is easy to become frustrated and disappointed if problems continue unsolved for very long.

Equipment will need continued reevaluation as your child grows older and larger. He may need an appliance with a larger capacity, or he may require a totally different product. Changes in equipment will probably be needed when he becomes a teenager and his skin changes, there is a weight change, or if his activities change significantly.

How to Manage the Equipment

After insuring you have the appropriate type of equipment, using the right technique in changing it is essential. The following is a suggested routine:

(1) Assemble all the supplies where they are handy. An empty box can be used to keep the supplies together. This can also be carried into the bathroom or wherever the change is to be made. In the beginning, it may be necessary to follow instructions, but later it will become second nature.

The supplies you will need depend on the type of appliance used; but in either event, you will require soap and water, wash cloth, and wick. If you are using a nondisposable, two-piece appliance, you will also need:

skin protection, barrier	adhesive tape or strips
adhesive disc	plastic retainer ring
faceplate	outlet valve
pouch	belt

If you use a disposable one-piece appliance, you will need the same items except for the faceplate, pouch, and plastic retainer.

(2) Wash your hands and the skin around the stoma with soap and water. Make sure the equipment is clean so that germs cannot grow within the appliance.

(3) Dry the skin around the stoma. Place a wick (rolled washcloth, gauze) over the stoma to prevent urine from leaking onto the skin after you clean and dry it. It is often a good idea to wait about two hours after drinking liquids to prevent the stoma from dribbling while changing the applicance. The first thing in the morning is often a convenient time to make the change.

(4) Apply skin protection or barrier. This may be a liquid or a solid sheet which is designed to prevent (or heal) skin irritation around the stoma. This is optional.

(5) Apply adhesive to the skin. This may be a liquid cement or a sticky disc. It is designed to keep the appliance attached to the body.

(6) If you use nondisposable equipment, place the faceplate over the stoma by centering it above the stoma first. Then quickly

remove the wick, lower the faceplate onto the skin and press firmly for a few seconds to help it adhere. Centering the faceplate or an adhesive ring takes practice. Place the wick back into the center of the stoma to continue absorbing the urine.

Pull the pouch over the lip of the faceplate. This may take more pulling if the pouch is new. Pull the retainer ring over the pouch.

If you use disposable equipment, remove the backing off the disposable bag. Center it over the stoma and press firmly.

(7) Place the adhesive strips or tape around the edges of the faceplate or disposable bag so the equipment will stay on longer. This will also make it possible for your child to swim or bathe with his equipment on.

Some children require more adhesives than others and you will find out only by experience.

(8) Be sure the outlet valve from the appliance is in the closed position and securely fastened.

(9) Fasten the belt. It should fit snugly enough to make a slight mark in the skin.

(10) Removing the equipment should be done gently. Empty the appliance first. For nondisposable equipment, unfasten the belt, and remove the plastic retainer ring. Separate the pouch from the faceplate. If it is time to remove the faceplate use an adhesive solvent or gentle traction on the skin. Do not pull the faceplate too hard because this can remove the top layer of skin and cause irritation. The adhesive disc will need to be removed from the faceplate with a solvent or with your fingernail. For disposable equipment, gently remove the appliance and discard it.

(11) After the equipment is removed, the skin should be thoroughly cleaned. The nondisposable pouch should be taken off daily and washed. A plain vinegar solution makes an excellent soak, and will remove any crusts. The faceplate should not stay on the skin longer than seven days. Commercial cleaning products are also available.

(a) It is a good idea to have two sets of equipment so one can be cleaned and aired while the other is worn. Also, when the pouches are rotated, they last longer.

(b) An appliance should be replaced when it becomes impossible to clean and the faceplate will not lie on a flat surface.

(c) Disposable appliances are especially useful for fostering cleanliness in children doing their own care.

(d) The pouch should be emptied when it is half full. Excess urine in the bag will place too much pull on the adhesive and tend to loosen it. A container should be used for emptying the bag if a bathroom is not available.

(e) A leg bag can be worn underneath clothing. Some children find it easier to store and empty urine from that position.

Other Types of Ileal Conduit Care

PSEUDO-EPITHELIOMATOUS HYPERPLASIA (LIKE "DISHPAN HANDS"). If the opening of the faceplate is larger than the stoma, the surrounding skin tends to be bathed in urine. Due to the constant irritation from moisture and chemicals in urine, a condition of wart-like bumps develops. These are tender to the touch. This can be corrected with the appropriate size equipment. A protective barrier worn underneath the faceplate will also promote healing. When this condition progresses too long, it may require surgical treatment.

ALKALINE URINE. Ideally, urine should be slightly acid. This is nature's way of keeping urine free of germs and odor. Nonacidic urine is called alkaline, and can be detected with a special acid-alkaline test paper. You may suspect alkaline urine when the urine has a strong odor or when there are white patches, bleeding or crusting around the stoma.

There are several ways to keep the urine acid or nearly so. The following are examples:

(1) Drinking plenty of water.
(2) Drinking cranberry juice.
(3) Avoiding citrus fruits and juices.
(4) Placing white vinegar (1/2 water and 1/2 vinegar) in the pouch at night to bathe the stoma with an acid solution.
(5) Medication, such as Mandelamine and ascorbic acid.

BLEEDING STOMA. Blood vessels are close to the surface in stomas, so a little bleeding should not be alarming. If, however, the bleeding does not stop, you should call your child's physician, or whoever is caring for the stoma.

MUCOUS IN THE URINE. The inner lining of the ileum or small intestine, from which the conduit was constructed, will shed bits of mucous occasionally. If the mucous becomes very thick, then your child should drink more water. If the opening of the pouch becomes plugged, a gentle squeeze should loosen it. There is a commercial product available which will disperse mucous if this is a persistent problem

SKIN IRRITATION FROM ADHESIVE PRODUCTS. Any irritation around the stoma should be treated before it progresses too far. It is easier for your physician to treat such problems in the early stages. Gentle removal of the faceplate and adequate cleansing are the major ways to prevent skin irritation. If irritation persists, be certain your child is not wearing the appliance longer than seven days. If it is worn too long, germs can grow under the moist adhesive and irritate the skin. If an allergy is suspected, then skin tests to various adhesive and protective products can be performed.

PERSISTENT URINE LEAKAGE AROUND FACEPLATE. This can be a distressing problem. The following are questions to ask if leakage is a problem.

(1) Does faceplate fit configuration of body for all activities (sitting, lying, crawling)?
(2) Is opening for faceplate the correct size (one-eighth inch larger than stoma)?
(3) Have other adhesives and products been tried?
(4) Are belts and supports being used?
(5) Is the bag becoming too full before emptying?
(6) Has the pouch been worn so long (over seven days) that it falls off due to the adhesive being too old?
(7) Has your child gained or lost weight?
(8) Has your child entered adolescence or is the skin becoming oily?
(9) Is his clothing or the belt so tight that urine cannot enter the pouch?

Helping Your Child with His Own Care

Generally, it is most desirable for your child to change his own equipment and take responsibility for it. This will give him an opportunity to master a function of his own body (staying dry), and relieve you of this responsibility.

Children who have an ileal conduit when they are seven and older can be taught immediately how to change their equipment. Children who have surgery at a younger age generally need their parents to assume this care initially. Often it simply seems easier and quicker for the parent to continue, rather than to teach a child how to do it for himself. There are the ever present demands of schedules to be met and children learn this task slowly. Other times, it is simply an issue of parents not believing their child can accomplish this task. This is understandable in light of the many things which parents of disabled children must do for them. However, you should look at teaching self-care at an appropriate age as an investment in fostering your child's sense of accomplishment and control over his bodily functions, and in saving your future time. Ironically, it is difficult to encourage self-care skills even when you want your child to be independent.

Sometimes, children seem to lack interest in learning how to care for their own ileal conduit. This is particularly frustrating for parents who want to promote independence. However, it is a rare child who appears "lazy" without some underlying reason. Usually children who appear to lack motivation have a general lack of self-confidence in their ability to do the job quickly or adequately, or they have a general lack of self-care skills.

These problems may be helped by remembering the following:

(1) Practice makes perfect. If you accept an imperfect effort at first, your child will be motivated to continue and will gain skill each time. His willingness to try is the important factor, and he needs your praise.
(2) Select a time when you are not rushed and can patiently wait if he is slow. Sometimes we are not aware of how we send unspoken messages to others. A tapping foot or watching the clock can nullify a spoken message to "take your time."
(3) One skill builds upon another. Ileal conduit self-care needs to be built on a foundation of other skills such as bathing and dressing. With each accomplishment comes the self-confidence which maintains motivation for the next project.

Emotional Support for Those Affected by the Surgery

The affects of this surgery are generally felt by the whole family. Therefore, acceptance and adaptation becomes an issue for the family and especially the child. A relaxed attitude from a family can give a child a lifetime basis for acceptance. There are several sources of help for those affected by this type of surgery:

(A) *Professionals.* Accurate information can eliminate misconceptions and fantasies about an ileal conduit. Professionals can also help you keep the stoma, conduit and appliance in working order. This will reduce stress.
(B) *Parents of other children with an ileal conduit.* Talking with someone whose child has had this type of surgery can relieve many concerns. It is reassuring to learn that you are not alone in having certain feelings. Either professionals or parent groups can help you contact other parents who have experience.
(C) *Self Help Groups.* Osteotomy associations are found in many cities. They are a more specialized gathering of people who have had ileal conduits or similar surgery. Although members of these groups generally do not have spina bifida, they can be most helpful.

As your child grows and reaches the teenage years, he will naturally be concerned with how his body looks (body image). Adjustment to a change, such as an ileal conduit, can be particularly difficult at this time. It can be accentuated with concerns about how it will affect the development of close personal relationships. Booklets offering advice on the subjects of dating and sexuality for those with an ileal conduit are available.

School officials also need information about the ileal conduit. In addition to your personal explanation, a booklet on this topic can be helpful. Such booklets are available. This can help their understanding of your child's needs for access to the bathroom and privacy. Your child may or may not explain the ileal conduit to his friends, depending on his wishes. Frequently, a simple explanation is helpful to decrease curiosity.

CHAPTER 18

SKIN CARE

CHILDREN with spina bifida often develop ulcers or other types of skin problems. Most of the skin problems they develop are related to a decreased ability to feel pressure, pain, or hot and cold in some portions of the body, usually the lower extremities. In the areas where feeling is normal, these problems do not arise. Sometimes secondary problems, such as excess weight or contractures also contribute to the chances of developing skin problems. Understanding the skin and the problems which can occur should help you to prevent many of them. The following are the most important types of possible problems.

Decubitus Ulcers (Bed Sores)

Decubitus ulcers or sores are areas where the skin has been lost. The skin loss may be associated with damage to deeper tissues also, and the bed sores thus vary in degree of seriousness. In the child with spina bifida, there are many factors which determine if such a sore will form. Understanding these factors will help you to avoid sores and also assist in treating them should they occur.

Pressure

Spina bifida has interrupted your child's ability to send messages to the lower portion of his body and return messages back to the brain from the nerve endings located in the skin and deeper tissues. For this reason, your child may be unaware that anything uncomfortable is happening to his body. Otherwise, he would automatically change his position to avoid continued discomfort or irritation to his skin and deeper tissues.

Bony areas such as the tail bone, hips, knees, ankles or rib cage are important areas where sores may form. These protruding areas have more contact with pressure or rubbing from bedding, clothes or equipment. Pressure on these points squeezes the skin, resulting in a decreased blood circulation to that area.

Circulation

Blood contains the nutrients which are necessary to keep skin and

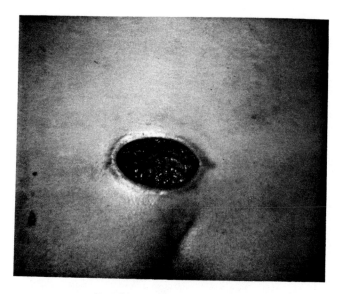

Decubitus Ulcer (over sacrum).

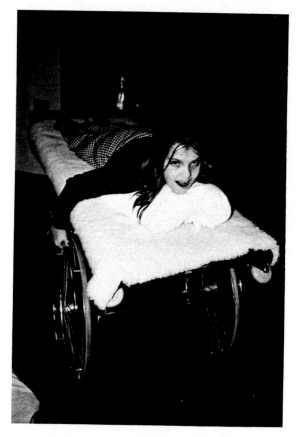

Keeping pressure off a decubitus ulcer on the buttocks.

PRESSURE AREAS

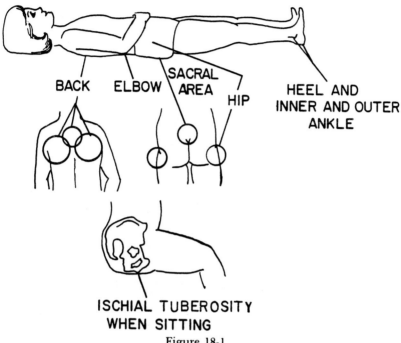

ISCHIAL TUBEROSITY
WHEN SITTING

Figure 18-1.

other tissues healthy. When the blood supply is decreased due to pressure, those areas which receive less blood become susceptible to injury. Children with decreased feeling generally tend to have sluggish circulation in insensitive areas of the body to begin with, and a further decrease can cause injury to the tissues. Once damage has occurred, it will heal slowly; since good circulation is also necessary for healing.

Nutrition

Good general nutrition keeps tissues and skin healthy, enabling the body to manage injuries better. Children with spina bifida are sometimes finicky eaters and may avoid foods rich in protein and vitamins (meats, fruits and vegetables) which help keep skin and other tissues healthy.

Moisture

A moist area is generally a comfortable environment for germs.

Moisture softens skin and causes it to crack and peel as well. This allows germs to enter deeper areas and can lead to infections.

Stages of Decubitus Ulcer Formation

Decubitus ulcers form gradually and usually go through predictable stages of development. It may be helpful to you to recognize each stage, then you can assess the severity of an ulcer and determine how it is improving or progressing.

Stage:

(1) Redness of skin.
(2) Redness with occasional blisters or skin breakdown.
(3) Layer of skin off, fat tissue below the skin exposed.
(4) Skin and fat tissue dead, muscle is visible.
(5) Skin, fat and muscle tissue are dead, bone is visible.
(6) All of the above tissues plus bone are involved.

Treatment

The treatment varies according to the stage of formation or the degree of tissue involved once a decubitus ulcer has occurred.

Stage (1). Relieving the pressure and gently massaging will increase blood circulation and the redness will disappear. If redness occurs after several hours in a sitting position, have your child lie down at home. If prolonged sitting at school results in these reddened areas, then obtain a cushion for his chair (foam, water). Rubbing the reddened area gently to increase circulation is helpful. Be sure your child's skin is as clean and dry as possible.

Stage (2). The redness will not disappear with rubbing, but may improve with relief of pressure. All the rules for Stage 1 apply here. Some people use material to toughen the skin and prevent it from breaking. Compound tincture of benzoin is satisfactory, but be sure your child does not lay on the area painted until it is completely dry. This compound sticks to many substances; and if the skin sticks to something unintended, your child may lose bits of skin when the two are separated. A light dusting of talcum powder over the area after it dries will prevent this. Ointments are not helpful protection and may even soften the skin and lead to further breakdown. A lotion applied with a gentle massage is better.

Stage (3). If the ulcer is small, it may heal with relief of pressure and the measures already mentioned. If your child is in school and the ulcer is in an area where sitting places pressure on it, then it is best for him to be on a small stretcher so that he will not sit at all. If this is not possible, a few days at home for close attention and care may save time and money in the long run. Be sure to keep the skin clean and dry to prevent infection from skin organisms. A mild soap and water should be adequate. Antiseptic lotions can injure delicate skin, and the alcohol content can actually burn the skin.

One simple method for drying and increasing circulation to the ulcer area is to use an ice cube and a hair dryer. Rub the ice cube gently over and around the area of the sore for approximately a half minute or until the area is cool to touch. Next, set the hair dryer for warm and wave it over the area for approximately five minutes at a distance of 12 to 18 inches, or until the area is warm. *Do not set the dryer on hot or direct the heat only at the sore area*, since this may damage the healthy skin around the sore. Repeat the ice and heat treatment two more times and then, if possible, use this treatment every two to three hours. You should see the area become dry and the damaged skin return to a pink and healthy condition.

Stage (4). The skin and fatty tissue are dead. You need to consult your doctor when this occurs because dead tissue must be removed before healing can take place. Your doctor may remove the dead tissue surgically, or he may direct you to use an enzyme product to do this. The enzyme will act only on dead tissues, but you must follow your doctor's directions closely to obtain the best results. Hydrogen peroxide may be used to remove dead tissue once it has been loosened by the enzyme. Your careful observations of what makes the sore better or worse will be needed in order to plan the best care.

Stage (5). The muscle tissue beneath the skin and fat is injured. The same measures will be required here as in Stage 4; but, in addition, surgery may be necessary.

Stage (6). The bone beneath the other tissues is also damaged. This depth of sore requires prolonged hospitalization, surgery, and often medication for infection in the bone.

THE BEST TREATMENT FOR
DECUBITUS ULCERS IS PREVENTION

Ammonia Burns

Ammonia from the urine can cause burns or blisters on the skin. When ammonia burns the skin, the appearance is similar to that following a mild-to-moderate sunburn. Ammonia occurs naturally in everyone's urine. When there is excess ammonia in the urine or it remains in contact with the skin, it can be quite irritating. When ammonia combines with moisture, it is even more irritating. Prolonged contact of ammonia with moist skin, such as occurs when a child is incontinent, can cause troublesome burns.

If your child has a urinary tract infection, bacteria in the urine will produce more ammonia than usual. Other germs that normally occur on the skin or in the stool can produce even more ammonia in the diaper and on wet skin. This aggravates ammonia sores even further. In addition, with a urinary infection, your child may wet more continuously than usual.

Soap and water is a safe and easy way to remove the urine and ammonia from the skin. Protecting the skin from irritation so that it can heal takes time and effort. Routine steps to prevent ammonia burns are:

(1) Change your child's diapers more frequently than usual when you suspect a problem. Consider paper diapers since fresh ones contain no germs. If you use cloth diapers, decrease the bacteria in them by soaking the diapers in diluted vinegar before washing or by adding Borateem™ or Diaparene™ to the water in which you rinse them.

(2) Protect the skin with a light coating of cornstarch. This keeps the skin dry and absorbs the ammonia. Do not use a large amount of cornstarch, as it becomes caked and difficult to remove.

(3) A light film of bland ointment such as Vaseline®, vitamin A and D, or Desitin® will protect the skin from irritation. It must be a light film, otherwise it will not be effective. Discontinue ointments and powders if redness and blisters develop, and wash with soap and water as often as possible.

(4) Try to find times when your child's skin can be dried and left exposed to the air without diapers.

Monilia

Monilia is a fungus and it commonly occurs in areas of skin which are moist and warm for prolonged periods. It is frequently found in skin folds and causes a characteristic fine raised red rash. Moisture and warmth are the main requirements for growth; therefore, continual wetting or stooling can give the fungus a good environment. Extra weight can cause increased skin folds and, thus, a place where the monilia can flourish.

Certain skin bacteria normally prevent the monilia from growing. If your child is taking antibiotics, this may change the type of bacteria usually found on the skin and allow the fungus to grow.

The same care as for decubitus ulcers and ammonia burns holds here. Clean skin and regular exposure to the air are the most helpful measures. If possible, avoid plastic pants at this time. Plastic pants retain both moisture and warmth. Antifungus medications such as Mycolog® ointment are helpful, but the problem usually recurs unless preventive steps are taken. Keeping skin folds and moist spots to a minimum by preventing or correcting excess weight gain is important.

Mottled Skin

Your child may have cool legs with patches of bluish coloring. This is called mottling and often occurs in children who have lost the sensation and motion in their legs. It is due to changes in circulation, but exactly why this occurs is not known. Mottling is not a problem in itself. However, the circulation changes which it represents signal that your child's limbs need to be guarded from sources of excess heat or coolness. Your child may not be able to feel when excess heat causes a burn or extra coolness results in frostbite. In addition, should burns or frostbite occur, the decreased circulation will make it harder for any damage to heal.

If your child should be hospitalized or have a cast on a leg, you should mention to the staff that your child's legs are usually cooler and bluer than average. This will help them to distinguish mottling from a cast which is too tight and needs to be loosened.

Your child may have an occasional skin problem. However, with careful checking and early treatment, most of these can be managed and prevent interference with the many activities which are so vital for a growing child.

Section III

Family Views of Children
with Spina Bifida

CHAPTER 19

PARENTS LOOK AT THE
EARLY MONTHS

OUR son, Stephen, who was born with spina bifida, is now nine months old. We hope that sharing some of our thoughts and feelings may help you know you are not alone. We hope, too, that it will help you to be optimistic for the future of your baby.

First, and foremost, we must express the deep love and great enjoyment Stephen has brought into our lives. We do have to admit, however, that we were overwhelmed when we found out he had this particular birth defect. Our hearts were filled with concern and uneasiness at what the future would bring and the problems with which we would have to deal. At first, it took much of the enjoyment out of having a new baby.

We had so many questions. "Would his limbs grow normally?" We were assured they would. "Would he be happy?" The doctors said it would be up to us and our attitude. And, as our questions were answered, some of our fears were erased.

The doctors were optimistic about his problems, and his general health was good. Their reassurance brought us peace of mind. The damage by the spina bifida was not the most severe type, yet certainly not a minor problem.

After the first couple of days passed, we were able to hold him; and finally, I was able to feed him. I was so anxious to get to know this beautiful, little person and give him the feeling of love and warmth that he so deserved. My husband found it a little more difficult than I, but I was the one who cared for Stephen. I offered my husband positive thoughts, and it wasn't hard to accept Stephen into our hearts.

It was difficult to leave Stephen at the hopsital when it was time for me to go home. Fortunately, I had my daughter at home to keep me busy. Also, I worried about her and leaving her each day when we visited Stephen at the hospital. I had been away for seven days for the C-section, and I did not want to leave my daughter any more than necessary. Therefore, we made our visits to the hospital nursery after her bedtime. If you have other children, you will be concerned about their well-being, too. It is important not to show more attention to one than the other. This can be especially difficult, since a new baby needs so much of your time and attention. A baby with spina bifida can require even more of your time, and there are doctor appointments and home exercises that the baby also needs. Knowing in advance that this may present a problem will be helpful in itself.

During the first several months, there may be many doctor appointments. It is so very important to your child that proper treatment start as soon as possible. I take Stephen to our local Birth Defects Center. My husband and I have confidence in the doctors and staff, and we are pleased with the care Stephen is receiving. With proper treatment, we are hopeful he will not have further complications or require more surgery than is necessary.

Our hope is for continued research to help children with spina bifida reach their full potential. Through our love and encouragement, we plan to give Stephen the strength and courage to try new feats. We are eager to help him accomplish all that he possibly can. The love and enjoyment Stephen has brought into our lives has far outweighed the concerns that we have had for him.

CHAPTER 20

LIFE IS MAKING THE MOST
OF WHAT YOU HAVE

Danny came into this world seven and one-half years ago to a mother who had an overwhelming feeling that something was going to be wrong. Fears became reality when the doctor announced in the delivery room that Danny was a boy with spina bifida. This started us on the road with our fifth child. Although this road may not have been as rough for us as it has been for other parents of children with spina bifida, it has not always been easy and has had its ups and downs.

Being a parent of a child with this congenital defect, it is important to know as much as possible about your child's disability. You should establish contact immediately with a primary physician who is *interested* in your child and who will be *responsible* for coordinating his total medical care. Parents should learn about spina bifida and the multiple problems associated with this defect. If at all possible, it is helpful to become associated with a spina bifida parent's group in your area.

Danny, who was operated on at the age of eight hours, is a happy, outgoing child in the second grade in the public school system today. His residual damage, due to the myelomeningocele, is a hypertonic, neurogenic bladder, which has resulted in urinary incontinence, absence of sensation around his buttocks, and bowel incontinence.

We have been working on bowel training since Danny was about four years old. Through encouragement and perseverance, we have him "bowel managed" about 95 percent of the time. He has an occasional accident, and this is usually associated with physical exertion (such as gym or play at home). Some of the things that helped us most in bowel training were a daily routine, regular schedule, and close attention to diet. We also used a mirror to show him what he could not feel. Lastly, and most importantly, we encouraged him. This is especially important when failures seem to outweigh the successes.

Danny's primary problem is urinary incontinence. He is presently on Ditropan®, which has enabled his bladder to relax more and stretch enough for him to void 200-300 cc in the morning and at other quiet times during the day. We are not this successful when he is playing, as he dribbles quite frequently when he is physically active.

He is an active child, and his ability to run and climb is nearly

237

normal. Although we notice some loss in his fine motor control, he is able to keep up with his peers. Sometimes he does complain that he is "it" much too often in games of tag, or that everyone beats him in running races in school. This fall Danny wanted to join an organized soccer league available in our area. I have to admit that he was very disappointed when we told him we would prefer that he not play.

The whole family loves to ski and, with a little fear in our hearts and encouragement from his doctors, we started Danny on the slopes three years ago. To our surprise, Danny took to skiing "like a duck to water" and today enjoys skiing from the very tops of the Vermont mountains.

Our main hope is that Danny will continue to progress as his environment expands. He accepts his "problems" (as he calls his disability) and has had only a few experiences where children have teased him. I think Danny is lucky to be part of a very close family and to attend a school where both the teachers and the nurse have been extremely cooperative.

We further hope that Danny will continue to grow and develop normally, and that his disability will become less of a problem. We want him to find his place in the world as a happy, useful citizen, well accepted by his friends and associates. As a friend said to me shortly after Danny was born: "Look around. Everyone is handicapped to some degree — either physically or mentally. No one is perfect. Your happiness and success in life is determined by making the most of what you have."

CHAPTER 21

FAITH AND INDEPENDENCE

WHEN Tonya was born, I was simply told "something is wrong with her spine." I was living in Georgia at the time, and it wasn't until we moved north years later that I heard the term spina bifida. Later it was explained to me by a local parents' organization, and I began to understand more fully.

At the time she was born, it did not seem that Tonya's problem was very serious. The doctors explained that her open spine was not serious and that treatment could help her. When she was moved to a large medical center in Georgia, I saw other children with more serious cases of spina bifida. At the same time, I learned that the severely paralyzed child who lived next door had been born with an open spine. Gradually, I learned more about the problems of the children who have this defect. I was thankful that Tonya's condition was not more severe.

My family was most helpful to me in those days. They were hurt and disappointed at having a grand-daughter with this problem; however, they did not let it show. They did not want to worry me, and they tried to hide their feelings. At the time, I did not realize how hard they were trying to be optimistic. This was fortunate, since I needed someone to show me what was good and right about my baby at that time. Possibly a large part of the reason they could be so encouraging was that they, too, did not accept that Tonya's case was very severe. This attitude was to our benefit. If the damage caused by her spina bifida had been worse, it would have been even harder in the beginning.

My mother not only offered me encouragement, but she showed me how to act with my baby. Tonya was my first child, and I was struggling with the normal aspects of baby care and also the problems of spina bifida. I tended to pity Tonya in those days, but my mother treated Tonya like a normal baby and later encouraged her to take care of herself as much as possible. I might still be pitying Tonya today, if my mother had not shown me that my daughter needed to be treated as normally as possible.

When Tonya was two years old, we moved to Rochester. The two of us living alone was frightening. However, I was fortunate to find an excellent babysitter who shared the responsibility of Tonya's care. Also, I must add that the Lord has watched over us. My faith in the Lord has helped me be independent and to care for Tonya all these years.

Tonya is nine years old now, and I have faith that things will go smoothly for her as she gets older. One of my worries at the moment is that she is physically developing but is not old enough to understand what it means. It is often difficult for her to understand and express her emotions and affections appropriately.

Many of the problems I have with Tonya are ones that I think would exist if she did not have spina bifida. However, I do get anxious when we are visiting a friend and she has an accident in her pants. It is embarrassing for both of us. She has had better bowel control over the last few years, but still needs constant reminding in order to avoid accidents.

In general, I do not think my life is any different than my friends. With the help of the Lord and the independence my parents encouraged me to have, Tonya and I are doing well. We have been eligible for welfare for many years, but have never depended on it. I want Tonya to experience and to value independence as she grows up. I want to provide Tonya the very best in life, and hope she will get a college education. Trusting in the Lord, I know she will reach her full potential.

CHAPTER 22

HELPING YOUR CHILD SUCCEED

$\mathbf{A}$S we tried to arrange some of our thoughts into a
meaningful discussion on being the parents of a disabled child, we
faced a problem. We knew some of our thoughts would be obvious to
those parents who have teenagers with disabilities. However, we were
hopeful that parents of newborns would also be seeking information
on the future challenges they would face with their child. For this
reason, we are going to be talking about many areas that may seem
obvious to some, yet appropriate for inclusion in a book of this type.

Let's begin with the following statement. Your child, who was born
with a birth defect, is not necessarily going to be a burden. However,
he will become a burden unless he receives the proper help and
backing from society and his family, and unless he has the proper
motivation from within himself. A disabled child is a *person* first and
disabled second. Remember also the pleas of most disabled people,
"Don't look at my chair or my crutches — look at me."

One of the first things parents of a child ready to enter school need
to do is formulate realistic goals for him. Early and complete educational screening and psychological assessment should be conducted to
assure an appropriately designed program to meet his needs. You
must know what potential your child possesses before you can work
out goals acceptable to both you and your child. Consult your local
school district for help. However, do not give up if you feel that you
are not getting the full cooperation of your school after making this
request. Most states have laws governing the provision of education
and supportive services needed by disabled children. Go to the handicap committee in your local school district, or the comparable committee in your area, and insist that these services be made available to
you and your child. Remember that this kind of educational guidance
needs to be a continuous process which can help him develop to his
maximal ability as a useful member of society.

Allow your child to experience all the normal developmental stages
of childhood. Promote all the experiences and interpersonal situations he may encounter within his physical limitations, because they
prepare him for adulthood. Let him crawl through a leaf pile with
the other kids. He can help build a snow fort and throw snowballs.
With his limitations in mind, let your child be a *participant* instead
of a spectator. If you expect your child to achieve normal adulthood
within the limitations of his disabilities, he must have the opportunity to experience all the social and emotional forces that are part of

241

"growing up." For example, all teenagers love to shop and be on their own. Suddenly we realized that our 13-year-old son had never been shopping alone. The solution for us was to locate a covered shopping mall that had about 70 stores under one roof. At first we gave him a small list, some money and about an hour and a half to shop. We asked him to meet us at the ice cream parlor. The first two trips were unsuccessful, because he found clerks ignored him and he was too embarrassed to ask for help. However, after six months and a shopping trip about every third Saturday, success came. We now drop him at the mall at 11:00 AM with a friend (sometimes a date). They shop, have lunch, tour the fun stores and sometimes see a movie. This is a good healthy eight hours away from Mom and Dad on his own.

Do not encourage dependency. A dependent child grows up to be a dependent adult. You won't live forever to care for him. As hard as it may be, gradually let go of your child. Insist that he become independent. One of the more gratifying experiences as parents of a disabled child is the day when your child achieves complete independence in a project such as dressing himself, when he tells you that he is going to the store alone in his chair, or when he tells you about his first date.

Many children will need encouragement to get enough courage to attempt these projects on their own. They will go through stages of "I can't do it." As a parent don't give up during this time, as your child's future independence is the result of a series of small successes through which he gains enough confidence to attempt a more difficult task.

How does this work? Here is an example of how our son gained the ability to go to the store independently:

(1) Talked to the police about wheeling toward traffic.
(2) Obtained a bike flag for chair.
(3) Practiced going up and down the road within sight of home.
(4) Planned the route and negotiated the curbs. (On the first trip to town, one parent went along.) NOTE: Do not assist, even if there are tears and swearing.

One year later, the goal was achieved! He now goes to town or to his friends and back. Do we worry? Of course! Do not let it show, however. If you are sure of his successes, he will be sure too.

Develop in your child or young adult a sense of pride through successful experiences, realistic responsibilities, and the feeling that he is loved as a capable human being. He may meet failures on a daily basis with physical barriers such as stairs, bathooms and curbs. Develop playtime games in which he is able to succeed. Assign chores that he is capable of completing successfully; such as setting the table, drying dishes, making a salad, and feeding the household pets. Give him the opportunity of being a "winner."

Help your child develop an understanding of the nature of his disability. As he grows, his natural questions relating to his disability offer you an opportunity to provide answers, simply and honestly. As time goes on and the questions become more specific, your answers can become more detailed.

A good understanding of his disability will also help your child deal with society's lack of understanding. Your child must learn to understand himself before he can accept himself and develop attitudes which will help make him acceptable to others.

How do you help him develop understanding, acceptance and a good attitude?

(1) Encourage your child to talk about his disability, anger and fears.

(2) Do not hide facts from him.

(3) Do not spare your child discipline you would normally give to your other children.

(4) Give him responsibilities.

(5) Encourage him to engage in activities normal for his age.

Do not underestimate the need for you and your child to have periods apart from each other. Families with children who have no disability benefit from a break in the routine. This "vacation" time for a family with a disabled child is even more important. Pressures do build and the time away will benefit both you and your child. Take advantage of the Handicapped Children's Camps sponsored in many communities by organizations such as the Rotary Club. These camps may be available on a no-charge basis to most disabled children and provide an experience that would normally be denied children with physical disabilities. Do not be ashamed of the feeling that you look forward to this time away from your child. It is natural and healthy. Your emotional health and your ability to be effective with your child can depend a great deal on these breaks.

Should your family have problems, do not blame your disabled child. Alcoholism, desertion, physical abuse, etc. would probably have developed as a family problem eventually, regardless of the presence of a special child. Maybe problems related to your disabled child enabled the family problems to manifest themselves sooner than they might have under different circumstances. Many parents turn to blaming their child, rather than admitting their own personal weaknesses. Sometimes unjust feelings of self-blame and guilt for your child's disability are at the base of conflicts. Unresolved, these can be costly to your emotional health and your marital relationship. This, in turn, can have an adverse effect on your children. It is hard enough to be a parent, but it is even harder to be the parent of a disabled child. Seek professional counseling for these difficult problems. Parent groups provide another type of support, although of a different nature.

Some of the well-known sources of help for you and your child are:

(1) Local Birth Defects Center or Spina Bifida Clinic.
(2) Local and State Rehabilitation Agencies.
(3) Youth and Family Services Agencies.
(4) National Crippled Children's Association.
(5) National Foundation — March of Dimes.
(6) Spina Bifida Association of America.
(7) Local Spina Bifida Association.
(8) Health, Education, and Welfare Agencies.
(9) National Easter Seal Society and its Local Organizations.
(10) Community Mental Health Clinics.
(11) United Cerebral Palsy Association.
(12) Mental Health Association.
(13) Association for Children with Learning Disabilities.
(14) Local Vocational and Technical Schools.

You may have the impression that our views are rather idealistic. You may feel that the ideas are good, but that your child is different and these suggestions will not work. Although you know your child better than anyone else, do not discard our suggestions without giving them a real try. Overlook the criticism you may get from others for your efforts.

We are idealistic, but also realistic. Our son is a fifteen-year-old and was born with severe spina bifida resulting in paralysis from the waist down and all the associated problems. He has had fifteen surgical procedures including shunts, an ileal loop, and many orthopedic operations. He is wheelchair bound. He is in regular school. He has been ridiculed and teased. He is afraid and often angry. He is also happy and laughs. He is often successful. He is a person, and we love him dearly.

CHAPTER 23

OUR DAUGHTER IS A FIGHTER

OUR daughter is fifteen now. She can best be described as a strong-willed girl . . . a fighter. It seems that nothing gets her down for long, even medical complications. I don't feel we taught her to be so determined about what she wants out of life. It is just her way. She is the kind of child who would even make what is wrong for her, right.

Thinking back, there may have been some incidents which influenced how she would turn out. The following affected us as parents and, in turn, changed how our daughter was treated.

One day when Cheryl was four, a physical therapist (Dean) came over to the house to discuss exercises. While we were talking, Cheryl's leg fell off her chair. I jumped up and put it back in its place. Dean told me that it was wrong to do things for Cheryl which she was capable of handling herself. Getting angry, I essentially threw him out of the house. Later, after talking to my husband about what happened, to my surprise he said, "I have been wanting to tell you the same thing." A week later, Dean returned and said jokingly, "Am I still allowed in the house?" I was still angry about hearing the painful truth, but in he came. If it had not been for him teaching me something for Cheryl's own good, I would still be "babying" our daughter.

There were other contributing factors to Cheryl's well-being. *First,* she has done many of the same things as the rest of the kids. She has shopped and gone to movies. Camp has been the single greatest experience for her. I would almost go as far as to say, "it has made life worthwhile." We were not missed when she was away and she told us it would be that way.

Through Cheryl's exposure with those at camp who were blind, deaf or retarded, she learned that some children have greater disabilities. Without this experience, she probably would only have stayed home and felt sorry for herself.

The exposure to 17 and 18-year-old counselors was also good. They can be more open than adults. It helped us to see how they could frankly explain to Cheryl how to behave without her falling apart. We were shown again that she was more durable than we thought.

Second, Cheryl has been disciplined the same as the other kids. Once she was spanked on her fanny, and she laughed and told us it did not hurt. She also told us that "You are not supposed to spank a paralyzed person." We found a spot on her arm which hurt and that

245

took care of that situation. By the way, we also took the consequences of her not talking to us and her saying, "You do not understand me."

There are not many things which have stood in Cheryl's way to being a typical teenager. The wheelchair is perhaps the most important thing, because it is so visible and is an ever present reminder of her disability. Right now, Cheryl is worrying about how it will affect her social life with boys. Those who take time to push her are suspect for their motives. She thinks they are doing it because they feel sorry for her. Hopefully, when she gets older, she will feel good enough about herself to sort out and accept those offers that come for the right reasons.

Cheryl's teen years are bound to contain some lack of self-confidence and painful moments. However, it is normal for teenagers to lack confidence and fall for others who do not return their affection. We see Cheryl's older sister going through the same things, and she does not have spina bifida. Parents have to remember that the teenage dramatics and trials are normal and that every rejection is not because of spina bifida.

Our expectations are that when Cheryl's teenage years are over, she will emerge more mature. Marriage is something we think she could handle, just like driving a car and having an apartment on her own. Cheryl is smart enough to make these things work. She has always seen the same things for herself as will be possible for her sister. For a long while, being independent will probably be more important than settling down. I think she would like first to discover what she can do with her life.

As far as girl friends go, they have taken her spina bifida in stride. Growing up with her has given them a chance to understand how she is special and how she is the same as they. When the girls have stayed overnight, they have been unaffected by her catheterizations and other procedures. It has always seemed that children are more accepting than adults.

Over the years, there have been other family members to consider as well. The children have certainly had to share more than they would have ordinarily. Our older girl has developed an interest in helping the disabled. Perhaps her interest and sensitivity has been a positive effect of having a disabled sister. One younger son has seemed to stick closer to us for a longer time. This may be because he did not share as much attention in the previous years. Right now his father is trying to spend more time with him. This is especially important for a boy.

It seems that fathers of disabled children, in particular, take a back seat in what is happening with their child. Generally, there are financial reasons to keep fathers working hard and away from the family. Sometimes the physical care needed by the disabled child may worry them and keep them from getting too involved. Most important is that fathers have less opportunity through the years to talk with others about their feelings and what is happening. All this may make it harder for fathers to adjust to the situation.

As parents of a teenager, we are currently dealing with some of the effects of our own aging. When your family starts to grow older and prepare to leave the house, it strikes you that your life is passing all too quickly. You naturally think about what you missed, and perhaps lash out at those who mean the most to you. At times families need to be as patient with the needs of parents, as with the needs of the children.

Whatever the parents' needs are for having their children around, they, nevertheless, have to push them to be independent. Your disabled child especially needs to be prepared for independence so he can manage when you are no longer there. If you start doing that from the beginning, you will feel more confident during the teenage years. Talking with someone along the way about your feelings can enable you to accomplish what needs to be done. It is unfortunate that it is so difficult to reach out for the very things we need most.

CHAPTER 24

MY PARENTS GAVE ME SELF-CONFIDENCE

I AM a 24-year-old male who was born with spina bifida and scoliosis. I spent the earliest part of my life in the hospital. There was never more than a two-year stretch at home until my teenage years. From what I understand, it was uncertain whether I would live until my fourth year.

Despite my health problems, school went well for me. I skipped the third grade and was mainstreamed around the sixth grade into a regular classroom. This was beneficial for me, since dealing with the disabled and nondisabled alike would be something I would experience all through life. However, when given the choice about high school, I selected a school which had provisions for the disabled (especially in the gym program). By attending this special high school, I did not have to develop new friends. Many of my classmates from grammar school were there, and this seemed to be an important consideration at that particular time.

In my second year in high school, I became active in wheelchair athletics and the Paralympics. As a matter of fact, I missed my high school graduation because of competition in the International Paralympics. Table tennis, weight lifting, and the 100-yard dash are my best sports. I have competed in these events for the international games. I have also been a competitor in the national games for the javelin, discus, swimming, shot put and quarter mile. Participation in sports has been an important part of my life. My current goal is to compete in the next Paralympics in Russia and retire to coaching afterwards.

After high school, I attended college and enjoyed the first year. However, the school was not particularly arranged for the disabled. They did not have a sports program in which I could participate, and this produced a lot of stress for me. The combination of personal pressures and the lack of school programs contributed to my becoming ill and leaving in the sophomore year.

Finding a job became the next task. I have held jobs as a bookkeeper for a department store, nursing home, and community center. However, I like my current job the best yet. I work with salesmen and telephone orders. At the time I was hired, my boss clearly wanted a qualified person; but from the beginning he was willing to consider a disabled person.

Some of the employment problems I have experienced are: physical barriers; complaints that I will be a fire hazard, or present insurance problems; and fears that I will be a poor health risk. Employers often feel the disabled person will have poor attendance or need extra assistance. Also, some employers expect to pay the disabled less on the assumption that "we are grateful to have a job." The biggest problem is getting an opportunity to show what we can do.

Three years ago I married a girl who was physically normal. We had a good life together until our divorce this year. It is hard to explain why our marriage ended, but I do not think my disability was a major factor.

The past 24 years have been most eventful. I attribute this success to several of my strong points. My *self-confidence* is one of them — I know that achieving within my realm is possible. *Self-control* is another — I do not fly apart when there is a problem. A *sense of humor* is undeniably the third.

There have been so many instances when humor has eased an uncomfortable moment. I can recall the time when a friend with spina bifida and I were traveling to some national games in New England. We had a flat tire, so I crawled out of the car and onto the ground to inspect the damage. It was not worth hauling my wheelchair out of the crowded back seat. As I lay on the ground, a police cruiser pulled up behind us. The policeman stepped out, walked over, and looking down at me said, "Are you a polio?" At that point he stepped up to the car. Peering at my friend he said, "My gosh, there's two of you!" It took a sense of humor to chuckle at his statement and see the situation through the policeman's eyes, but we both managed to laugh.

On that same trip, we stopped at various restaurants along the way. We would unpack only one wheelchair to save time and trouble. That meant one of us had to ride in on the other one's lap. That attracted a few stares, but we certainly provoked them. On one occasion a waitress came over and inquired, "Where are you going?" We replied, "To a convention called Cripples Anonymous. It's a group like alcoholics anonymous. If you feel like a cripple, you call us up and we talk you out of it." You would be surprised at the people who believed we were serious.

My favorite gag is the reply to the ever present question, "What's wrong with you?" Depending on how gullible my friends and I think the inquirer is, we might reply, "I have spine-o-lio. It is a cross between spine problems and polio, and you catch it from eating margarine."

Although humor has been helpful to me, I have been told that sometimes it can be a defense against other emotions. That is something that must be kept in proportion.

Speaking about emotions raises the issue of the social scene for a young man with spina bifida. It is awkward for a disabled man in a wheelchair to approach a physically normal woman and begin a conversation. This is largely because she may not quite know how to respond to you. It can be done, however. You simply have to pull up your suspenders and give it a try. Something like, "I know I can't dance, but would you like to talk for awhile?", usually works. Also, striking up conversations in class is helpful. The secret to it all is self-confidence. On a date you must expect to have a good time. If you enter any situation with a defeatest attitude, you will end up defeated.

Many people through the years have been instrumental in helping me develop into what I am today. Teachers who have spent special time with me, the family minister, and friends have all been an important part of my life. However, without a doubt, my parents have played the most significant role and have been my greatest inspiration. They have been with me all the way.

Primarily, they gave me confidence in myself. They let me explore just like any other child. Certainly they were concerned about my safety, but they were not overprotective. They realized that a child is a child, regardless of any disability. Also, the efforts of my parents to maintain a close family was a source of strength for me.

My parents helped me to understand my medical condition. This is essential if a child is to care for himself when he gets older. They explained my limitations but, at the same time, established a routine of caring for myself. These early habits have aided me in becoming an independent adult. Now my doctors communicate directly with me about my condition. This helps me handle the situation better, and I can use a logical approach to solving my problems.

Parents probably commit most of their errors in overprotectiveness, because they are afraid for their child. At the root of this fear is a lack of understanding about their child's condition and his needs. I have a friend who has cerebral palsy. He wants to separate from his family, but I know it will be difficult for him to be an independent adult and care for himself. Unless he can learn to care for his own needs, it may lead to a tragic situation when his father and mother are no longer around. Parents need to exert every effort to encourage independence in their children. That is why a local Birth Defects Center and a book such as this are important. Parents need encouragement, information, and help all along the way when their child has a special problem.

CHAPTER 25

BECOMING AN INDEPENDENT ADULT

WHEN children with spina bifida become adults, they start thinking, as do most young adults, about finding a job, getting an apartment, and starting a life of their own. Then, perhaps they might consider getting married, buying a house, and starting a family of their own.

The opportunities available to your child with spina bifida to lead an independent, productive life as an adult, are plentiful. Great strides have been made to erase the skepticism which for centuries plagued the world as to the disabled person's ability to become a useful citizen. Fortunately, for all the disabled, the world has finally come to realize that many of us can be independent if a few phycical adjustments (wider doorways, ramps, elevators, etc.) are made to schools, apartment buildings, and places of business. Helping us become independent also reduces the financial burden on taxpayers. Hopefully, when your children become adults, they will be able to seek employment and have their own apartments or houses without too much worry about architectural barriers. Of course, some barriers exist and perhaps always will. But, even now, if you look hard enough, you can usually find what fits your particular needs.

Strides have also been made to remove the psychological barriers toward disabled persons. This is especially true with employers. Employers, in most cases, are concentrating on the ability rather than the disability of the individuals they hire. Of course, some people still have the tendency to become nervous and skeptical when confronted with a person in a wheelchair, or someone who uses braces and crutches. It is in these instances that the adult with spina bifida, or any person for that matter, must make a special effort to do a good job. Actually, the situation is much better today than years ago; because, when given the chance to prove their abilities, statistics have shown that the disabled person is, in most cases, a more reliable worker and has a better attendance record than most co-workers who have no disability.

Your child will no longer feel dependent upon you as parents to transport him to and from work and to social activities when he has his own transportation. Learning to drive and buying a car are big factors in gaining one's independence. There are rehabilitation centers which provide driving lessons for the disabled and offer advice as to the best type of car and hand controls for each individual. This is especially important if the person is paralyzed from the hips down.

251

Obtaining insurance for the car may present a problem, since some insurance companies still consider disabled persons a great risk. Of course, you can usually find an insurance company which realizes that the disabled driver is generally more careful than most other drivers.

The next phase of gaining independence is finding an apartment or house. Here you may encounter architectural barriers. Most individuals prefer not to live in a hospital situation, where almost everything seems really too convenient. In selecting a place to live, it is essential that a disabled individual in a wheelchair be able to enter a building independently. This requires a smooth, flat entrance or a ramp. In apartment complexes, where there is only one step into the building or perhaps a curb, it is easy to construct a small ramp. This can be done at little cost, and will allow the disabled person to enter the building or go over the curb without any assistance. Some things to look for within the complex are narrow doorways (especially into the bathroom) and low cupboards (it is impossible to reach high cupboards from a wheelchair). Also, make sure the laundry facilities are accessible.

Physical independence is a very precious thing to a disabled person and is something that should not be denied to anyone. Parents must teach their children to compensate for any physical inconveniences and to live their lives to the fullest. You must teach your child to be self-confident, to believe in his abilities, and not to worry about his disabilities. If your child with spina bifida is able to gain self-confidence and make a contribution to society, you as a parent can be very proud. It is your guidance and encouragement that will help determine if he will be able to succeed as a useful citizen.

Section IV

A Story For Children

Sue Stone's Guitar Recital

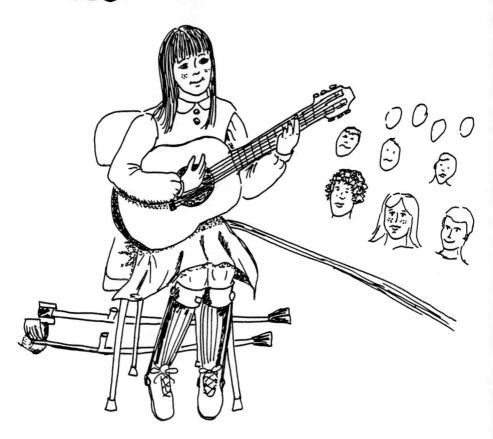

Figure 1.

SUE STONE'S GUITAR RECITAL

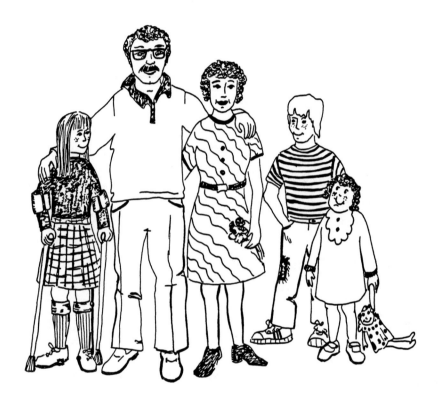

Figure 2.

SUSAN STONE is nine years old. Like a lot of nine-year-old girls, she has long brown hair and blue eyes. Her eyes twinkle when she laughs — which is often, because she likes jokes and funny stories.

Susan has a mother and father, a twelve-year-old brother, Bob, and a six-year-old sister, Jenny. She has two grandmas and a grandpa. Susan's family lives in a city in a brown house, where Susan has a bedroom of her own.

Susan is in the fourth grade at her school. She likes school because there are lots of kids and lots of new books to read in the library. She likes school, too, because she is learning to play the guitar.

One day Susan had a guitar lesson after school. She took the late bus home. When she got off the bus, the kids in the neighborhood were playing baseball. They asked her if she would like to bat.

"No thanks. I have to practice for the recital Firday."

Susan started up the walk to her house. She was in a hurry. She wished she could run like other kids, because she wanted to tell her Mum what her guitar teacher had said . . . She was the best guitar player in the fourth and fifth grades.

Susan couldn't run because her legs do not work well. She wears braces and uses crutches. She has spina bifida. (Say it spy-nuh biff-id-uh). It happened to her when she was a baby, before she was born. A place on her spine did not form right. It turned into a bump. Nobody knows why it happens to some babies and not to others. Doctors do know it is nobody's fault. It just happens.

When spina bifida happens to a baby, the nerves inside the bump on the spine do not grow right. Nerves are like telephone cables, only they are not made of wires. They carry messages back and forth between places in the body and the brain. In spina bifida, the nerves below the bump are not formed right. They cannot carry messages like normal, healthy nerves.

It's like this: Susan can think in her head about moving her leg, but much of the message cannot get past her spina bifida to her leg. So her leg only moves a little bit. Also, if her leg or foot gets cut and tries to send the message "Ow, I got cut," the message never reaches Susan's brain. She cannot feel the cut. Maybe you think it would be great not to feel a cut, but it's dangerous. If you do not know you are stepping on glass, you could cut your foot before you noticed anything was wrong.

So Susan cannot walk fast or run. It took her a long time to go up the walk and get into her house. Susan barely had time to wash up before dinner. She liked dinner time at her house. Everybody told what had happened that day. Her Dad usually told them a funny story about where he worked or a joke.

Susan did not feel hungry. She did not feel like talking much. Her mother noticed she was not eating.

"Susan, is everyting ok? You like sphagetti and you have hardly touched it."

"I'm ok. Just tired I guess."

"How did practice for the concert go?" asked her Dad.

All of a sudden, Susan felt very sad and lonely. Her eyes got full of tears. Next thing she knew, she was crying hard and talking at the same time. "I'm the best guitar player in the fourth and fifth grades."

Her Dad said, "Something must be bothering you. Can you tell us what it is?"

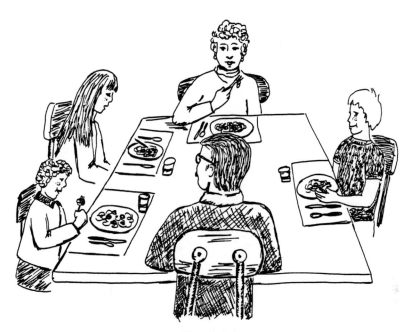

Figure 3.

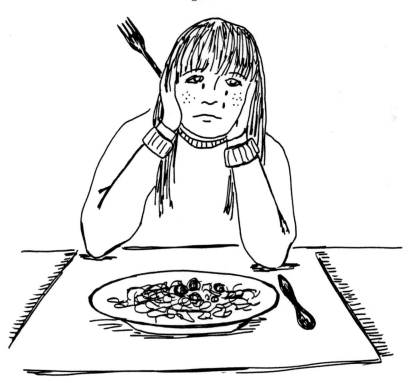

Figure 4.

Susan's crying stopped and a lot of talk came pouring out. She was scared about the guitar recital, not about playing the guitar, but about climbing the five steps to the stage. It takes her *so* long to climb steps and everybody will be watching. They might think, if she cannot get up the stairs, she probably cannot play the guitar either.

Susan started feeling sad all over again. "Maybe I ought to drop out of the recital. Nobody will want to wait while I climb up the stairs."

"Susan, you could drop out you know," said her mother. "But remember how hard lots of things were the first time you did them alone? . . . dressing yourself, climbing on the regular school bus, catheterizing yourself . . . and now you do all those things so well."

Her Dad said, "Susan, think it over. Is it really going to be too much for you? Do you think if you and I practiced a bit in the auditorium when it was empty, you would feel better about playing in the recital?"

Susan did not answer for a minute. "Daddy, I'm tired. I will think about it tonight and tell you at breakfast. I'm all mixed up right now."

After dinner, Susan did her homework and undressed for bed. When she was in the bathroom catheterizing herself, she remembered the many things she had already learned how to do.

Spina bifida made it hard to do some things which most people learn easily. When she was little she had to work harder to stand up alone, to walk straight, and to climb up stairs. Going to the toilet was harder too. Because doing these activities is harder for kids with spina bifida, Susan learned to use special helps like braces and crutches and to take special trips to the bathroom.

Susan cannot feel in her feet and legs. She also cannot feel when she needs to go to the bathroom to urinate or to move her bowels. Susan used to dribble and make messes. She used to wear diapers which made her feel like a baby. She hated them.

Last year when Susan was eight, she stopped wearing diapers. She learned to take herself to the bathroom. She goes every three hours, starting as soon as she wakes up in the morning.

Susan cannot feel when her bladder is full of urine. She also cannot send a message to her bladder to let the urine go. So she has learned to empty her bladder using a catheter (say it KATH-it-ter). Susan's catheter is a soft plastic tube about as long as a drinking straw. It's just about as thick. (A boy's catheter is longer, but the same thickness.) It is made up of soft plastic. Susan has learned how to gently put her catheter up inside herself in the hole where her urine comes out. The catheter tube lets her urine trickle out into the toilet. That way it doesn't get trapped inside her.

Susan lay in bed remembering. She felt half sad and half happy. She liked being able to catheterize herself and ride the regular bus and go to a regular school. She was glad she did not still go to the special school.

She began to remember that at the special school there were no stairs. But then the' special school did not have guitar lessons or recitals either. She really liked playing the guitar. She guessed she liked the guitar more than she minded everybody watching her climb the stairs. She decided to practice climbing them with her Dad.

The next afternoon Susan and her Dad practiced going from her seat to the steps, up the steps, and across to her chair in the middle of the stage. After many tries, she got her time down to three minutes. Her Dad said if she started right when the clapping started it would seem like less time.

The next night she was washing for dinner when she heard her Grandma Black in the kitchen say to her mother . . . "But Esther, that's too hard for poor little Susan to be in a program with normal children. In my day we never expected crippled children to do such things. The poor child should just be loved. It's not right. It's not fair to her."

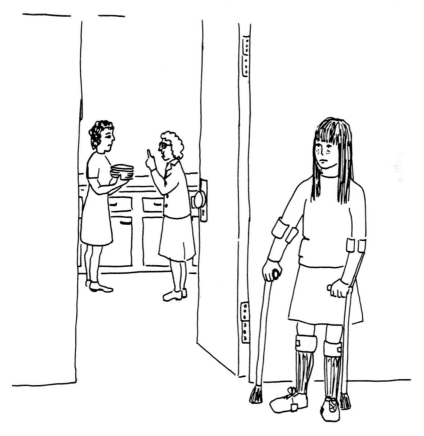

Figure 5.

She thought, maybe Grandma Black is right. It is too hard going up those stairs with everybody watching. Grandma understands. She never makes me help with dishes and stuff like Mom or Grandma Stone do.

Susan shut the bathroom door to catheterize herself. She did not hear her mother say, "Things have changed today. Sure it's hard for Sue. But she *can* do it."

That night in bed Susan thought some more about hard things that had happened because she had spina bifida. The new neighbors had kept their kids out of her yard, because they thought spina bifida was catching!

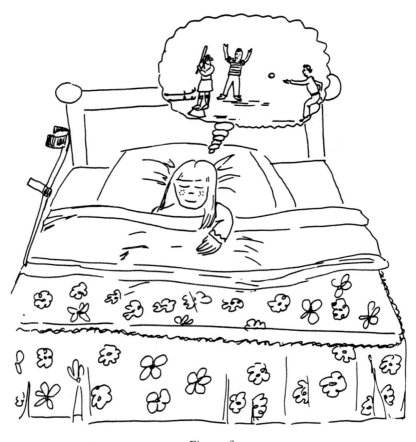

Figure 6.

She thought how impatient her brother got when it took her too long to put her braces on — how he'd push her hands away and say in an angry voice, — "Hurry up, Dummy, you're so slow."

Susan sometimes remembered feeling sad when the neighbors' kids ran off to do things like roller-skate and ride a bike, which she could not do. But then, she remembered, she could do some things they could not do, like "pop wheelies" in a wheelchair. She almost always wins Indian wrestling matches, because her arms are very strong from pushing her crutches. Susan loves baseball. She goes to bat and then someone runs for her. She can really hit the ball. She likes playing outdoors a lot, but she likes indoor games too, like checkers and Monopoly®. She likes to win.

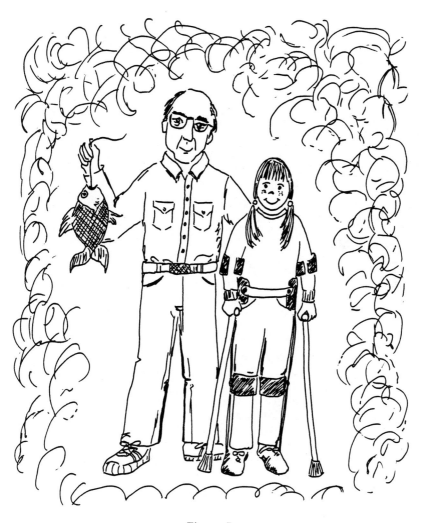

Figure 7.

Susan lay in bed and felt sorry for herself. Very sorry. She thought about other things that bother her about spina bifida. People who do not know her often stare at her. They make her feel like making a freak face at them, but she does not do that. Her mom said people stare because they are interested and want to understand.

Susan used to think she had spina bifida because she had bad, angry feelings sometimes and was a bad person. Her Dad told her everybody has angry feelings sometimes and not many people have spina bifida. . . . so bad feelings do not make spina bifida.

Susan was getting sleepy and a bit bored with feeling sad. She thought about the camping trip she had with Grandma and Grandpa Stone. Grandma Black had been very upset and kept telling Susan's mom it was too hard for Susan to go to a campground. Why they did not even have flush toilets, and "Poor dear Sue could catch cold sleeping in a tent." Susan remembered that she had a wonderful time rowing and swimming. She had not caught a cold but she did catch a fish. Grandpa cleaned it, and Grandma showed her how to cook it over a fire. She did have to do the dishes for breakfast as her chore, but Grandpa dried and sang songs while they worked. One night he woke her up to watch shooting stars over the lake. She would never forget hearing a loon's call break the stillness of the night.

All of a sudden Susan decided. Maybe she was not the fastest walker in the recital, but she was the best guitar player. She was going to play! She wasn't going to drop out. Her molasses-legs were going to climb those stairs so her fingers could play! She fell asleep chuckling to herself, "Molasses-legs."

The night of the recital arrived. Susan's seat was at the end of the first row. She and Lissa McNab talked and watched everybody enter the auditorium and fill all the seats. They waved to their families. Finally, Mr. Snodgrass, the principal, came onto the stage and started to talk. All the people in the auditorium hushed. He welcomed everyone and introduced the music teacher, Mrs. Jones.

Susan's stomach felt like it was full of butterflies — all flying in different directions. It felt awful.

José Gonzales played his drums. Everybody clapped. Marcia Horwitz almost ran up the steps to the stage and played her clarinet. She did not squeak once, and everyone clapped again.

Susan watched as her turn got closer and closer on the program. Susan's solo followed Michael Washington's trumpet piece, and she hoped it would never end, but it did. She grabbed her crutches and stood up. She started toward the steps to the stage. Mrs. Jones put her guitar on a chair at the center of the stage. It looked a mile away.

Susan counted each time her crutches clumped, 3, 4, 5. The auditorium was so quiet. 6, 7, 8. "Why are my hands so wet?" 9. 10, 11. "Come on, molasses-legs." 12, 13, 14. "Maybe they're quiet because they think I'll fall. But I won't." It seemed a year until she reached the chair and dumped her crutches. Mrs. Jones had helped her tune the guitar. Her fingers started to play.

She played her piece better than ever before. When she ended, everybody clapped and clapped. Her brother even whistled! She bowed and smiled, picked up her crutches and started off the stage. It did not seem very long before she was back in her seat. Lissa smiled, leaned over and whispered "Nifty" to her.

There were five more pieces after Susan's. At the end the audience stood up and clapped. The performers all stood up, turned around and bowed back.

Susan felt good. She had really played well. She was very happy she had decided to play in the recital. It was funny. . . . . somehow her molasses-legs did not really matter so much any more. Her fingers worked just fine, especially playing the guitar!

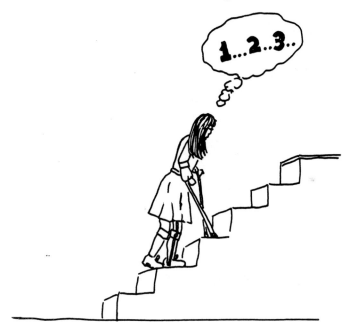

Figure 8.

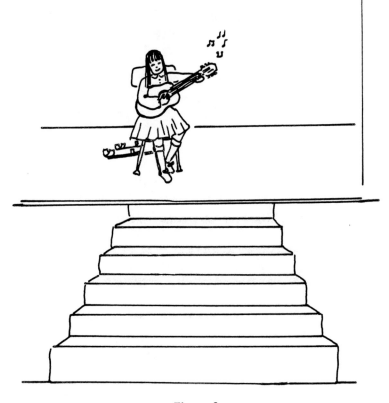

Figure 9.

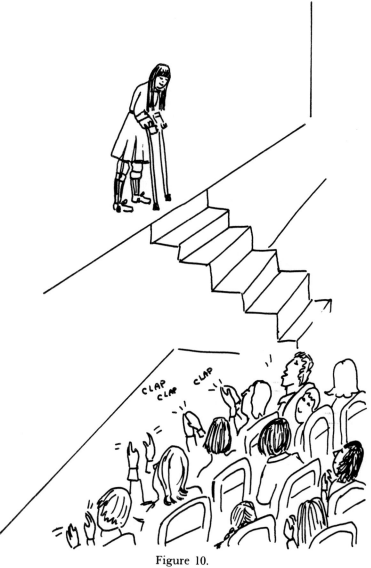

Figure 10.

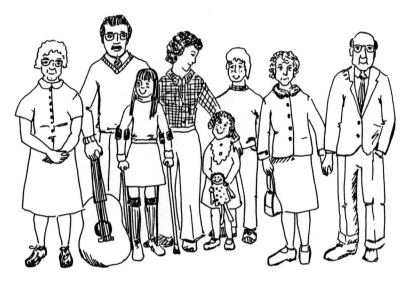

Figure 11.

Appendices

A. Helpful Readings on Spina Bifida
B. Organizations That Might Be Useful
C. Equipment Needed for Home-Care After Spine Surgery
D. Bradford Frame (building instructions)
E. Using the Parapodium
F. Mealtime Suggestions to Assist in Bowel Control
G. Glossary

HELPFUL READINGS ON SPINA BIFIDA AND DISABILITIES

BOOKS

Swinyard, Chester B., Ph.D., *The Child With Spina Bifida*, 1975
Institute of Rehabilitation Medicine
New York University Medical Center
400 East 34th Street
New York, New York 10016
    Booklet describing spina bifida and some of the procedures for treatment.
Henderson, Maria and Synhorst, Diane, *Care of the Infant with Myelomeningocele and Hydrocephalus: A Guide for Parents*, 1975
University of Iowa
Iowa City, Iowa
Apgar, Virginia and Beck, Joan, *Is My Baby All Right?*, 1973
Pocket Books — Division of Simon & Schuster, Inc.
630 Fifth Avenue
New York, New York 10020
    Includes the cause and effects of birth defects, spina bifida and hydrocephalus.
Heisler, Verda, *A Handicapped Child in the Family, A Guide for Parents*, 1972
Grune and Stratton, Inc. — Division of Harcourt Brace Jovanovich, Inc.
111 Fifth Avenue
New York, New York 10003
    Deals with the feelings of parents as they attempt to cope. Written by a psychotherapist who was disabled by polio when she was a child.
Anderson, Elizabeth M. and Spain, Bernie, *The Child With Spina Bifida*, 1977, Methuen and Company, Ltd.
Love Publishing Company
Denver, Colorado 80222
    An excellent overview of the social, emotional, educational, and intellectual aspects of children with spina bifida.
Gordon, Sol, *Living Fully: A Guide for Young People with Handicaps*, 1975
Ed U Press
Charlottesville, Virginia 22902
Gordon, Scales, and Everly, *The Sexual Adolescent* (Communicating with Teenagers about Sex), 1979
Duxbury Press
North Scituate, Massachusetts 02060

McDonald, Eugene, M.D., *Understand Those Feelings,* 1962
Stannix House, Inc.
3020 Chartiers Avenue
Pittsburgh, Pennsylvania 15204
  Suggestions for parents of disabled children on how to deal with their children, professionals, society and themselves. Discusses the usual feelings and thoughts of parents.
Spock, B. and Lerrigo, M., *Caring for Your Disabled Child,* 1965
Collier Macmillan Paperback Division
Crowell Collier & Macmillan, Inc.
866 Third Avenue
New York, New York 10022
  A general coverage of ways to care for a disabled child.

PERIODICALS

Accent on Living
P. O. Box #726
Gillum Road and High Drive
Bloomington, Illinois 61701
  Quarterly magazine with articles pertinent for those with various disabilities and the important people in their lives.
The Exceptional Parent
Psych-Ed Corporation
264 Beacon Street
Boston, Massachusetts 02116
  A bimonthly magazine for guiding parents of special children. A practical approach.
The Pipeline (of the Spina Bifida Association of America)
104 Festone Avenue
New Castle, Delaware 19720
  Contains national news and recent developments of importance to those affected by spina bifida.

READINGS ON CHILD DEVELOPMENT AND PARENTING

Brazelton, T. Berry, *Infants and Mothers: Individual Differences in Development,* 1969
Brazelton, T. Berry, *Toddlers and Parents: A Declaration of Independence,* 1974
Dell Publishing Company
750 Third Avenue
New York, New York 10017
  Uses brief ancedotes as examples. Shows normal development and typical problems faced by all parents. Explains how to deal with them. *Infants and Mothers* covers the first year, month by month. *Toddlers and Parents*

deals with ages one to three. Discusses issues of importance to single or working parents.

Dreifurs, Rudolph, M.D. and Stoltz, V., *Children: The Challenge*, 1964
Hawthorn Books, Inc.
260 Madison Avenue
New York, New York 10016
Discusses dealing with children in a practical way. Emphasizes helping the child develop his own sense of responsibility.

Frailberg, Selma H., *The Magic Years*, 1959
Charles Scribner & Sons
597 Fifth Avenue
New York, New York 10017
Discussion of first five years of a child's life with examples of how children experience situations and learn to cope with them. This book helps parents understand their child's behavior by seeing how it looks from their child's viewpoint.

Gesell, A., Ilg, F., and Ames, L. B., *Infant and Child in the Culture of Today: The Guidance of Development in Home and Nursery*, 1974
Harper and Row Publishers, Inc.
10 East 53rd Street
New York, New York 10022
Covers the behavior and typical day of children at various stages between birth and five years. Discusses guiding children's behavior. There is a chapter on nursery school behavior and lists of suggested toys and play materials, books for children and selected readings.

Ginot, Hiam G., M.D., *Between Parent and Child*, 1965
Avon Books, The Hearst Corporation
959 Eighth Avenue
New York, New York 10019
Offers suggestions for dealing with problems and situations such as discipline, sex, education, independence and anger in childhood and adolescence.

Gordon, Thomas, M.D., *Parent Effectiveness Training: The Tested Way to Raise Responsible Children*, 1975
A Plume Book, New American Library
1301 Avenue of the Americas
New York, New York 10019
Explains techniques for improving quality of the parent-child relationship. This technique is sometimes taught in workshops.

Salk, Lee, M.D., *What Every Child Would Like His Parents To Know*, 1973
David McKay Company, Inc.
750 Third Avenue
New York, New York 10017
Straightforward question and answer format offering practical advice to parents about emotional issues of early and mid childhood.

READINGS ON INFANT STIMULATION AND PLAY

Beck, Joan, *How to Raise a Brighter Child*, 1967
Trident Press, Division of Simon & Schuster, Inc.
630 Fifth Avenue
New York, New York 10020
  Activities and games to help toddlers and young children increase their
  awareness of the world.
Gordon, Ira J., *Baby Learning Through Baby Play*, 1970
St. Martin's Press, Inc.
175 Fifth Avenue
New York, New York 10010
  Games and activities for fun and stimulation, developing a sense of
  security, self-esteem and intellectual growth. For newborn to two-years-
  old.
Gordon, Ira J., *Child Learning Through Child Play*, 1972
St. Martin's Press, Inc.
175 Fifth Avenue
New York, New York 10010
  Fun games and activities for developing intellectually and physically. For
  ages two to four years.
Gregg, Elizabeth & Boston Childrens' Center Staff, *What To Do When
There's Nothing To Do*, 1968
Dell Publishing Company
750 Third Avenue
New York, New York 10017
  Play ideas using materials available in the home for two- to six-year-olds.
  Lists good books, records for children and readings for parents.

READINGS FOR CHILDREN

Rockwell, Harlow, *My Doctor*, 1973
Macmillan Publishing Company, Inc.
866 Third Avenue
New York, New York 10022
  An illustrated portrayal of a child's visit to a female pediatrician.
  Portrays the use of stethoscope, blood pressure cuff, tongue depressor, eye
  chart, scales, reflex hammer and syringe. There is no particular
  discussion of feelings.
Scarry, Richard, *Richard Scarry's Nicky Goes to the Doctor*, 1971
Western Publishing Company, Inc.
1220 Mound Avenue
Racine, Wisconsin 53404   Ages three to six years
  Mr. Scarry's books are popular with children and his description of
  Nicky's visit to the doctor for a check-up is thorough. It is attractively
  illustrated.

Walde, Gunilla, *Tommy Goes to the Doctor*, 1972
 Houghton Mifflin Company
 1 Beacon Street
 Boston, Massachusetts 02108
   A description of an examination by a pediatrician during which the
   doctor and the mother help Tommy deal with his feelings.
Schima, Marilyn, *I Know a Nurse*, 1969
 G. P. Putnam Sons
 200 Madison Avenue
 New York, New York 10016   Ages two to three years
   A second grade class is given an explanation by the school nurse of the
   roles of nurses in many situations. There is some description of hospital
   experiences included.
Deegan, Paul and Larsen, Bruce, *A Hospital: Life in a Medical Center*, 1970
 Amecus Street, Inc. Affiliate of Creative Educational Society, Inc.
 Box #113
 Mankato, Minnesota 56001   Ages four to seven years
   A thorough description of the many departments of a large hospital.
Falk, Ann Marie, *The Ambulance*, 1966
 Burke Publishing Company, Ltd.
 73 Six Point Road
 Toronto 18, Ontario, Canada   Ages three to nine years
   A well-illustrated book about a five-year-old boy's emergency appendec-
   tomy and his natural reactions to the experiences involved.
Froman, Robert, *Let's Find Out About the Clinic*, 1968
 Franklin Watts, Inc.
 845 Third Avenue
 New York, New York 10022   Ages Kindergarten to three years
   Describes roles of hospital clinic personnel and the procedures used.
Hass, Barbara S., *The Hospital Book*, 1970
 John Street Press
 1315 John Street Park
 Baltimore, Maryland 21217   Ages four to ten years
   Gives a realistic picture of hospitalization, since it includes the unplea-
   sant as well as the pleasant sides of the experience. The illustrations
   include some of bones and organs.
Andry, Andrew and Schepp, Steven, *How Babies Are Made*, 1968
 Time Life Books
 New York, New York
   Beginning sex education with brief, easily understood explanations and
   attractive illustrations.

BIBLIOGRAPHIES OF INTEREST

Spina Bifida Association

Library — Spina Bifida Association of America

P. O. Box 6-1974
Elmhurst, Illinios 60126
  For further reading about the care, recreation and education of persons
  with spina bifida, there is an excellent bibliography of books, pamphlets,
  magazines and handouts compiled by the Spina Bifida Association of
  America.

Easter Seal Society

The National Easter Seal Society for Crippled Children
2023 West Ogden Avenue
Chicago, Illinois 60612
  Have bibliographies and handouts of articles of interest to the disabled
  and their families.

National Foundation

National Foundation — March of Dimes
800 Second Avenue
New York, New York 10017
  Have lists of publications, films and exhibits available to those interested
  in the disabled and their families.

United States Government

Superintendent of Documents
  U. S. Government Printing Office
  Washington, D. C. 20402
    Selected government publications on disabilities available. If you are on
    the mailing list, you will receive notice of new publications as well as
    those already in print.
DHEW Publication No. (HSA) 74-5402
"Books That Help Children Deal with A Hospital Experience" by Altshuler
  U. S. Department of Health, Education and Welfare
  Public Health Service
  Health Services Administration
  Bureau of Community Health Services
  5600 Fishers Lane
  Rockville, Maryland 20852
  A bibliography of books for children about health-related experiences.

ORGANIZATIONS THAT MIGHT BE USEFUL

Aid to Adoption of Special Kids
3530 Grand Avenue
Oakland, California 94610
   Aid to potential adoptive parents of children who are difficult to place.
Academy of Dentistry for Children
1240 East Main Street
Springfield, Ohio 45503
American Academy of Orthotics and Prosthetics
1444 N Street, Northwest
Washington, D. C. 20005
   Certified Professional Practitioners
American Wheelchair Bowling Association
Don Pinault, Executive Director
2424 North Federal Highway, Suite 109
Boynton Beach, Florida 33435
American Nurse's Association
2420 Pershing Road
Kansas City, Missouri 64108
   Professional organization of registered nurses.
American Occupational Therapy Association
6000 Executive Boulevard, Suite 200
Rockville, Maryland 20852
American Academy of Pedodontics
211 East Chicago Avenue
Suite 1235
Chicago, Illinois 60611
American Association of Mental Deficiency
5201 Connecticut, Northwest
Washington, D. C. 20015
   Interested in general welfare of retarded.
American Orthotic and Prosthetic Association
1444 N Street, Northwest
Washington, D. C. 20005
   Firms and individuals who manufacture orthoses, limbs, etc.
American Physical Therapy Association
1156 15th Street, Northwest
Washington, D. C. 20005

American Public Health Association
1015 18th Street, Northwest
Washington, D. C. 20036
Professional organization with interested consumers to promote personal and environmental health.

Association for Children with Learning Disabilities
5225 Grace Street
Pittsburgh, Pennsylvania 15236

Association for Children with Retarded Mental Development
902 Broadway
New York, New York 10010
Parents and professionals interested in retarded children and young people.

Association for the Care of Children in Hospital
Box H
Union, West Virginia 24983

Association of Rehabilitation Facilities
5630 Wisconsin Avenue
Washington, D. C. 20015
Rehabilitation Centers in the United States and Canada.

Big Brothers
220 Suburban Station Boulevard
Philadelphia, Pennsylvania 19103
Volunteer laymen who under professional supervision give guidance through friendship.

Big Sisters
135 East 22nd Street
New York, New York 10010

Council on Adoptive Children
302 Leslie Street
Lansing, Michigan 48912
Concerned about hard-to-adopt children.

Council of World Organizations Interested in the Handicapped
122 East 23rd Street
New York, New York 10010

Division on Physically Handicapped, Homebound and Hospitalized
School of Special Education and Rehabilitation
University of North Colorado
Greely, Colorado 80639
Educators and those involved in services to physically handicapped.

Easter Seal Home Service
185 Madison Avenue
New York, New York 10016

Goodwill Industries of America
9200 Wisconsin Avenue
Washington, D. C. 20014
Concerned with employment and training of disabled.

Indoor Sports Club
    1145 Highland Street
    Napoleon, Ohio 43545
        Social and Recreational Club for Disabled.
International Association for Enterostomy Therapy
    1701 Lake Avenue, Suite 470
    Glenview, Illinois 60025
International Mailbag Club
    3641 Marydell Place, Apt. 4
    Cincinnati, Ohio 45211
        Brings cheer to shut-ins with letters and cards.
International Society for the Rehabilitation of the Disabled
    120 East 23rd Street
    New York, New York 10010
        Clearinghouse for distribution of books and material.
Just One Break
    373 Park Avenue South
    New York, New York 10016
        Helps place disabled in employment situations.
National Association of Children with Learning Disabilities
    4156 Library Road
    Pittsburgh, Pennsylvania 45234
National Association of Mental Health
    1800 North Kent Street
    Rosslyn, Virginia 22209
        Citizen's voluntary organization devoting itself to the fight against
        mental illness.
National Association for Retarded Citizens
    2709 Avenue E East
    Arlington, Texas 76011
        Parents and professionals interested in the retarded.
National Association of the Physically Handicapped
    76 Elm Street
    London, Ohio 43140
        To advance social, economic and physical welfare of the disabled.
National Association of Physical Therapists
    P. O. Box 367
    West Covina, California 91793
National Committee for Prevention of Child Abuse
    111 East Wacker, Suite 510
    Chicago, Illinois 61601
        Stimulates greater public awareness.
National Congress of Organizations of the Physically Handicapped
    7611 Oakland Avenue
    Minneapolis, Minnesota 55423
        Organizations of physically disabled assist other organizations with their

programs and structure.

National Council for Homemaker — Home Health Aide Services
67 Irving Place
New York, New York 10003

National Easter Seal Society for Crippled Children and Adults
2023 West Ogden Avenue
Chicago, Illinois 60612
  Conducts various programs for physically disabled.

National Foundation March of Dimes
Box 2000
White Plains, New York 10602
  Goal is to prevent birth defects through research.

National Genetics Foundation
9 West 57th Street
New York, New York 10019
  Sponsors nationwide network of genetic counseling and treatment centers.

National Paraplegia Foundation
333 North Michigan Avenue
Chicago, Illinois 60601
  To inform and educate medical professionals.

National Rehabilitation Association
1522 K Street North West
Washington, D. C. 20005

National Wheelchair Athletic Association
Benjamin H. Lipton, Chairman
40-24 62nd Street
Woodside, New York 11377

National Wheelchair Basketball Association
Stan Labanowich, Commissioner
101 Seaton Building
University of Kentucky
Lexington, Kentucky 40506

National Wheelchair Softball Association
Dave Van Buskirk, Commissioner
P. O. Box 737
Sioux Falls, South Dakota 57101

Spina Bifida Association of America
3435 Dearborn Avenue, Suite 319
Chicago, Illinois 60604
  Parents and professionals devoted to educating the public about spina bifida and improving life for individuals with spina bifida and their families.

United Ostomy Association, Incorporated
111 Wetshire Boulevard
Los Angeles, California 90017

World Association to Remove Prejudice Against the Handicapped (WAR PATH)
Drawer H
Pearsall, Texas 78061

EQUIPMENT NEEDED FOR HOME-CARE AFTER SPINE SURGERY

1. *Hospital bed* with overhead frame. The need for this depends on the size of your child and the firmness of the mattress on his regular bed. It will be easier for you to care for your child if the height of the bed can be raised. This will prevent you from bending over while tending to his needs. A mattress which is too soft will not adequately support the healing spine. Beds are available through Home-Care Associations, hospital supply rentals and local loan closets.

2. *Mirrors* which can be attached to the overhead frame will allow your child to view television from a flat position. These are not readily available but are of great help to entertain the immobilized child.

3. *A trapeze* can be connected to the overhead frame. It can be grabbed by your child so he can assist you in turning him. This would have to be checked first with your orthopedist to determine if your child's back is ready for this kind of movement.

4. *Spectacles* are constructed like prisms. They will allow your child to look around without lifting up. They are useful for reading and TV watching and are available from the Public Library and opticians.

5. *A bedpan* is essential and the only practical method of evacuating while immobilized. A "fracture pan" type of bedpan is preferable, since it will slip under your child more easily.

6. *An over bed table* or similar item is a convenient place on which your child can rest his meals, books, games, and other items.

7. *Extra pillows* are helpful for propping your child on his side.

8. *Plastic pads* to place under your child will protect the sheets and mattress from soiling by stool or urine.

9. *A bell* or other means of getting attention is essential for safety.

10. *Bandages, dressings and medications* may be needed depending on the individual situation.

APPENDIX D

GUIDELINES FOR BUILDING AND USING A BRADFORD FRAME

Bradford Frame

To help prevent soiling of hip spica casts.

A Bradford frame can be built at home in any size, The usual sizes are:

13 × 30 inches
16 × 42 inches
18 × 50 inches

When building a frame, make sure it is large enough that the child's head is not resting on the bar.

Materials

The frame can be made of piping or wood.

(a) If using pipe, four square conduit pipe joints will be necessary and of the same diameter as the piping.

(b) If wood is used, the corners can be nailed or bolted in place.

Canvas or denim can be used for the material. The material should not be stretchable. There should be enough material to go around the frame with four to six inches to spare.

Metal eyelets (28) for canvas.

Rope

Two pieces of foam rubber, (one inch thick and the width of the frame ↘ the length of the frame less the size of split in the middle).

Heavy plastic sheeting to cover foam and canvas.

Materials Needed

Two pieces of electrical conduit piping ___ inches.
Two pieces of electrical conduit piping ___ inches.
Two pieces of canvas
28 metal eyelets
Rope, 1/4 inch
Two pieces of foam rubber, one inch thick ___ × ___
Heavy plastic sheeting to cover foam and canvas.
Plywood 1/4 inch (size of mattress)
Blocks or books — to elevate head of the frame.
Straps or rope to secure frame to ends of bed.
Plastic sheeting to protect center area.

To fit your child's crib.

To fit frame

280

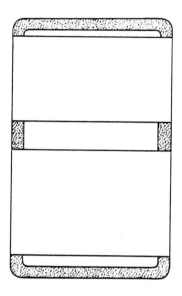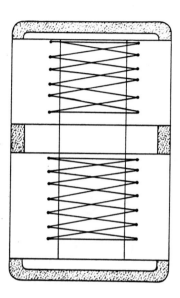

Construction

Make a rectangle using the four pieces of pipe or wood. Fit corners into joints or bolt and tighten.

Fold two- or three-inch seam over ends of canvas. Punch seven holes in either side and place eyelets in these holes. Place two pieces of canvas over frame and lace with rope. Make canvas as tight as possible.

Place the foam pieces over canvas. Cover with plastic and tape in back. You may want to cover each piece of foam with plastic, then cover with a pillow case and tape in place over canvas.

Setting up the Frame

Place a plywood over the mattress, this will protect the mattress. Elevate the head end of the frame at 30°-40° angle with blocks or books.

Strap or tie the frame at both ends of the bed.

Insert plactic sheeting over bedboard under the split in the Bradford frame.

Placing Your Child on Frame

The top of the perineal cut out in your child's cast should be just below the bottom edge of the top frame cover.

If necessary your child may need to be strapped to the frame to prevent sliding.

Keep sides of crib up at all times.

Caring for Your Child

Tuck plastic around the groin and buttocks area to protect the cast. A bedpan can be placed on the bed, below the buttocks, to catch urine and stool. In this way diapers can be kept off periodically.

Change your child's position at least every two hours during the day. Turn him onto his stomach frequently. When turning him, be certain that his toes do not hit the mattress.

Care of the Frame

Check the canvas daily. Prevent sagging by tightening the ropes as necessary.

Wash the plastic cover with soap and water if it becomes soiled. To cover the canvas and foam sponge pads, you may find it convenient to make sheets to fit.

Change linen daily and as necessary.

APPENDIX E

USING THE PARAPODIUM

Now that your child has received his parapodium, the time has come to begin the work which is necessary for a good start. The following training plan is designed to help your child learn the new tasks required for the effective use of this new brace. Keep in mind that any plan is only a guide and must be adapted to your child's special needs.

The First Week

Your child's body and mind will need time to become adjusted to the standing position. For this reason, the first week your child will be given what might be called a wearing schedule. This schedule increases the time your child is in the brace slowly to allow for his adjustment to standing. A sample schedule is as follows:

First day:
    1. Wear brace 15 minutes.
    2. Out one hour.
    3. Back into brace 15 minutes.
    4. Repeat throughout day.

Second day:
    1. Wear brace 25 minutes.
    2. Out one hour.
    3. Back in 25 minutes.
    4. Repeat throughout day.

Third day:
    1. Wear brace 35 minutes.
    2. Out one hour.
    3. Back in 35 minutes.
    4. Repeat throughout day.

Each day your child should wear the parapodium an additional five to ten minutes every time he is in the brace, until he is able to wear it most of the day.

MEALTIME SUGGESTIONS TO ASSIST IN BOWEL CONTROL

Breakfast

The day should start with
(1) Fruit juice, preferably prune or apricot.
(2) Whole wheat or granola bread or toast or ceral (Raisin Bran™, Bran Buds™, or some other cereal your child will eat, to which you should add one to two teaspoons of raw bran).
(3) Eggs as child desires.

Lunch

(1) Include a fresh or cooked leafy vegetable such as lettuce or spinach.
(2) Glass of milk.
(3) Meat, peanut butter and jelly, or tuna fish with celery sandwich.
(4) Fresh fruit if possible, as this increases the fiber content (orange, apple with skin, etc).

Supper

(1) Include potato or starch substitute (sweet potato, yams, macaroni, spaghetti).
(2) Meat or other protein source (cheese is constipating).
(3) Salad or cooked leafy vegetable.
(4) Fresh fruit if possible.
(5) Yellow or orange vegetable.
(6) Glass of milk (8 oz. maximum).

Snacks

Popcorn, high fiber cookies, nuts, sunflower seeds, and dried fruit. The use of bran or whole wheat in the diet is essential. Bran (unprocessed miller's bran) can be sprinkled over dry or cooked cereal; mixed with juice, applesauce, or yogurt; and added to soups, stews, or ground meats.

Foods to Stress

Fruits	*Vegetables*	*Cereals*
Apples (with skins on)	Carrots — raw	Heartland™
Peaches	Lettuce	Granola
Pears	Celery	Raisin Bran
Plums	Cauliflower	Shredded Wheat™
Berries	Radishes	All Bran™
Pineapple	Cucumbers	100% Bran Flakes™
Grapes	Tomatoes	
Nectarines	Green Peppers	*Cookies*
Apricots	Onions	Raisin Bran
Prunes	Broccoli	Oatmeal Marmalade
Dried fruits	Asparagus	Oatmeal Molasses
Oranges	Baked Potato with skin	
Grapefruit	Corn	
Raisins	Peas	
	Popcorn (with hulls)	

Foods Which May Be Constipating

Milk, cheese, bananas, chocolate.

GLOSSARY

ADL, Activities of daily living
  Ordinary tasks that we do every day (eating, dressing, climbing out of bed, bathing, etc.)
Abduction
  Movement of an arm or leg away from the body.
Acting out
  The behavioral expression of hidden emotional conflicts, such as the hostile feelings seen in various kinds of neurotic behavior.
Adduction
  Movement of an arm or leg towards the body.
Adductor release
  An operation that releases the adductor muscles in the thigh so that the leg can be moved away from the body.
Alpha-Feto-Protein
  A protein which the fetus makes and which is present in excess quantities in the amniotic fluid and blood of mothers who are carrying a fetus with an open spina bifida.
Ambulation
  The ability to move about independently. In contrast to walking, braces, crutches or extra equipment may be required.
Amniocentesis
  Procedure to remove amniotic fluid from around the unborn baby in the mother's uterus. "Alpha-feto-protein" in the fluid indicates that the baby may have spina bifida.
Amniotic fluid
  The fluid that the baby floats in within the mother's uterus.
Amniotic sac
  The thin sac which surrounds the baby and contains the amniotic fluid while the baby is in the mother's uterus.
Anal sphincter
  The muscle at the end of the rectum which allows one to control when bowel movements are passed.
Anencephaly
  A severe birth defect in which the brain is poorly developed and not covered by skin or bone. These infants die before or soon after birth.
Arnold-Chiari malformation
  An abnormal development of the brain which occurs in many children with spina bifida.

285

Arteriogram
    Special X-ray procedure to see blood vessels. It requires that a dye be put into an artery so that the network of arteries can be visualized upon X-ray. Sometimes done to see the blood vessels in and around the brain.

Anterior
    Used when describing something relatively in front of some other part of the body, e.g. the chin is anterior to the ear.

Arthrogryposis
    A birth defect where one or more joints (usually in the arms or legs) are not properly formed and allow little or no movement.

Attending Physician
    The physician ultimately responsible for the patient's medical care in the hospital.

Audiologist
    A specialist who tests hearing and determines when a hearing loss or other similar problem is present. Also, involved in selecting, fitting adjusting, and monitoring equipment to aid hearing.

Benzoin
    Brown liquid that leaves a sticky surface on the skin. Used to help bandages or ileal loop equipment stick better. Sometimes used to toughen skin.

Beta trace protein
    A protein found in the cerebrospinal fluid. When a fetus has spina bifida, this protein can leak into the amniotic fluid where it can be measured. Its value in prenatal detection is unclear presently.

Bladder
    The muscular walled sac that holds urine before it is passed to the outside.

Bilateral
    Both sides.

Bowel
    The intestine. Includes large and small intestines and rectum.

Body image
    The mental picture one carries of one's body, i.e. thin, fat, beautiful.

Braces
    Metal, leather, plastic and other materials built into a structure to support a part of the body.

Bradford frame
    An apparatus constructed of metal piping and canvas which will support a child in a spica cast. It helps prevent urine and stool from soiling the cast.

Brain Scan
    Procedure that uses a very small amount of radioactive material injected in the arm vein to show normal and abnormal parts of the brain.

Brain Wave
    See EEG.

Caries
    Cavities in the teeth.

Caster cart

Low toddler chair with wheels that allows the paralyzed child to move himself around by pushing on the wheels.

CAT scan (computerized axial tomography)

Special x-ray procedure. A computerized painless test that gives an excellent picture of the brain and the spaces in and around it.

Clean intermittent self-catheterization

A method of reducing urinary tract infections and contributing to urinary control in some children with a neurogenic bladder. Child routinely empties bladder by inserting a clean catheter into it.

CVP, Central venous pressure

The pressure of the blood just as it returns to the heart. It is measured through a long thin tube placed in an arm vein. Used after major surgery to monitor fluid needs and administer fluids and medications.

CSF, cerebrospinal fluid

The fluid that bathes the brain and spinal cord.

Cerebral arteriogram

X-ray procedure where dye is injected into an artery to outline the blood vessels in the brain. Abnormal changes in the brain that affect blood vessels can be seen.

Cervical area

The top section of the spine which is found in the neck.

Colace

A prescription medication to help soften the stools.

Comprehensive care

Health care that tries to deal with all the areas of need (medical, social, emotional, daily management).

Constipation

Inability to easily pass stools that are large and hard.

Contracture

A tightening of the muscles or ligaments which limits the movement about a joint. It occurs about joints when they are not used.

Coordinated care

Where the various specialists work together so that the child and family receives the most organized care possible.

Corner chair

Special chair that looks like a corner. The sides provide some support so that children with poor balance can sit more easily.

Counseling

Giving advice or support on how to cope with certain problems. Attempts to guide a person to reach their own solutions to problems.

Credé's maneuver

Applying gentle firm pressure on the bladder to force the urine out.

Cystometrogram

Procedure done by urologist that measures the pressure needed within the bladder before it will empty.

Cystoscopy

Procedure where the inside of the bladder can be seen through a tube passed through the urethra.

Cystourethrogram
X-ray study where dye is placed in the bladder through a catheter and the structure of the bladder and urethra studied.

Decubitus ulcer
An errosion of the skin and deeper layers of tissue from pressure and rubbing.

Denial
A defense mechanism in which the existence of intolerable actions, ideas, wishes, impulses and effects are unconsciously denied.

Dietitian
A specialist who can help you achieve good nutrition through proper food selection.

Disability
A bodily impairment which limits the execution of some tasks and skills.

Diarrhea
Loose watery stools which are passed frequently.

Disclosing solution
A solution which colors plaque on teeth so that it can be easily seen.

Dislocation
When a joint is displaced so that the bones forming it are not properly arranged.

Ditropan®
Prescription medication that may help those with a neurogenic bladder hold urine longer.

Dorsiflexion
To bend upward at a joint.

Dulcolax®
Prescription medication that can be given orally or by suppository and helps push stool out of the body.

Dwyer procedure
Name of the type of spinal fusion operation which is done to the anterior part of the spine. It requires surgery opening the chest.

Ejaculation
The ejection of fluid with sperm from the penis.

EEG, electroencephalogram
Nonpainful test that measures small amounts of electrical current arising from the brain.

EMI scan
A type of CAT scan.

Endotracheal tube
Plastic tube that can be placed in one's windpipe to assist breathing with a respiratory machine.

Enema
Fluid placed in the rectum to loosen stool and cause a bowel movement. Different types of fluid can be used.

Enterostomal therapist
Professional trained in the care of patients who have urinary or bowel diversion surgery (ileal loop, colostomy).
Ephedrine
Prescription medication used sometimes to help children hold their urine longer.
Erection
When the blood vessels in the penis become full of blood and the penis becomes larger and tense.
Extension
The act of straightening out a limb or part of body.
External sphincter
The outer muscle of the rectum which normally is under voluntary control and holds back the passage of stool until the individual wishes to release it.
Family Counselor
A trained lay person who supports parents under stress through listening and suggestions. Familiar with community resources and works closely with the social worker.
Family practitioner
A physician who cares for all the members of a family. Usually refers patients to a specialist when an unusual problem arises.
Femur
The large bone of the upper leg.
Fetoscopy
New procedure that allows obstetricians to see the unborn baby inside the uterus through a special instrument.
Fetus
An infant before birth, while still in the mother's womb.
Fissure sealant
A material which seals tiny cracks in the surface of teeth and thus helps prevent decay.
Flaccid
Limp and without strength or meaningful movement.
Flexion
The act of bending, especially at a joint.
Flexion release
An operation that releases the muscles which cause flexion of a limb and prevent extension.
Forearm crutches
Special crutches that are supported by the forearms.
Gastro-colic reflex
The normal urge to have a bowel movement after eating a meal.
Gastroenterologist
A physician who treats problems associated with the bowel and digestive system. Helps children with spinal bifida in prevention of constipation and bowel continence management.

Genes
The material in the body cells which carries the genetic information and characteristics to be inherited from parents.

Genetic counseling
Discussion with a specialist to determine the chance of a birth defect or other health problem occurring or recurring in a family. May include discussion of prenatal detection of birth defects.

Germ cells
The primitive cells which mother and father contribute to form a baby. Female germ cells are called eggs and male germ cells are termed sperm.

Gibbus
The bump which sometimes occurs on the back of the child with spina bifida when the vertebra are formed in a certain improper manner.

Grice procedure
The name of a surgical procedure that improves ankle function by joining bones together.

Guerney
A stretcher on wheels. A patient lying on the stomach can move it by pushing the wheels.

Habilitation
To develop an individual's functional ability and help him reach a more healthy condition. Differs from rehabilitation in that the individual is not regaining a lost ability.

Halo-femoral traction
Method of straightening the spine. A metal ring around the head is connected to pins through each thigh bone (femur) by rods. The rods can be lengthened by screws and force the attachments further apart thus stretching the spine.

Halo hoop
Refers to a general method used to help straighten the spine. The term includes halo-femoral and halo-pelvic traction.

Halo-pelvic traction
A method to straighten the spine. A metal ring around the head is connected to pins through the hip bones by rods which can be lengthened. Works in the same manner as halo-femoral traction.

Harrington rod
Metal rod which is connected to the spine during an operation to correct spinal curvature and provide extra support.

Heel cord lengthening
Surgery done on the heel to lengthen the heel cord when it is too tight and will not allow enough foot movement.

H frame
A bar placed between crutches so that they form an H.

House officer
A doctor in training in the hospital. Includes both interns and residents.

Hydrocephalus

A condition where the spaces (ventricles) inside the brain become larger than normal. The fluid within the spaces is usually under pressure.

Hydronephrosis

Condition of the kidneys where blockage to the outflow of urine causes the kidney to enlarge. Can lead to kidney damage.

Ileal conduit

A surgical procedure which creates an artificial urinary system. A section of small bowel (ileum) is connected to an opening on the wall of the abdomen. The ureters from the kidneys are connected to the other end of this bowel which then acts as a passageway for urine.

Impaction

A large amount of firm, hard stool lodged in the lower bowel that is difficult to pass.

Incontinence

Lack of control, usually referring to the passage of urine or stool.

Incontinence pants

Pants which are a cross between a diaper and regular underwear. Often used when a child is too large for diapers.

Inheritance

The passing of certain characteristics from parents to child through genes, i.e. hair color, size, diseases.

Intensive care

Hospital care in a special unit with extra equipment and personnel for those who are seriously ill.

Internal sphincter

Inner muscle of the rectum which controls the passage of stool into the lower bowel and rectum. This is not normally under voluntary control in anyone.

Intravenous

Medications or fluids injected into a vein with a needle.

IVP, intravenous pyelogram

X-ray study where dye visible on X-ray is injected into the vein and circulated through the kidney. This helps show some types of kidney damage or other related problems.

Kidneys

Two organs located inside the abdomen on each side of the lower back. They act to filter waste products from the blood, conserve body fluid, and regulate blood pressure.

Kondremul®

Prescription medication to help soften stool.

Kyphosis

An arch of the spine producing a bump or hump on the back.

Lateral

To the side.

Laxative

Medication or food which stimulates stool to pass through the bowel.

Lazy eye
When one eye does not look at the same object as the other eye.
Learning disability
Any difficulty in learning. Usually refers to problems in one or two areas of learning, such as with hand-eye coordination. Does not include mental retardation.
Ligaments
Strong tissues which connect two bones or a bone and a muscle.
Localizer cast
An adjustable cast to help correct curvature of the spine.
Lofstrand crutches
Special crutches supported by the hand and lower arm.
Lordosis
An arch of the spine which increases the hollow in the back, and makes the buttocks more prominent.
Lumbar area
The lower part of the back between the hip bones.
Lumbar spine
An area of the spine which is in the small of the back.
Lumbar puncture
A procedure to evaluate the cerebrospinal fluid. A needle is inserted into the lumbar spine to remove a small amount of fluid.
Magical thinking
A child's special way of looking at certain events, for example, believing that death is a temporary situation.
Meningitis
An infection in the cerebrospinal fluid.
Meningocoele
A type of spina bifida which affects primarily the coverings around the spinal cord.
Metamucil®
A nonprescription barley extract. Assists bowel movements by providing bulk.
Methylcellulose
A nonprescription medication which adds bulk to the bowel movements.
Monilia
A type of fungus that grows in moist places such as the mouth or diaper area. It is easily treated.
Multidisciplinary
Made up of many specialties, such as a team consisting of various types of doctors, a nurse, a social worker, physical therapist, etc.
Myelomeningocoele
A type of spina bifida which affects the spinal cord and the coverings around it, as well as the bones and skin.
NG tube, nasogastric tube
A thin rubber tube placed through the nose, down the throat and into the

stomach. It is often used after an operation to remove stomach contents and prevent vomiting.

Nervous system
A general term used for all of the nervous tissue in the body. This includes the brain, spinal cord and nerves.

Neural tube
The nervous tissue in the developing baby which starts in the form of a tube and then develops into the brain and spinal cord.

Neural tube defect
Any variation from normal in the development of the neural tube. Spina bifida is one example.

Neurologist
A medical doctor who specializes in problems which affect the nervous system.

Neurosurgeon
A surgical doctor who specializes in operations which involve the nervous system.

Neurogenic bladder
A bladder controlled by nerves which do not work properly. The nervous tissue triggering the bladder may be too active or not active enough.

Nurse
A health specialist who functions in different capacities, depending on the setting. Provides ongoing care and management of daily problems. Also, works with other health team members and parents in determining the type of treatment your child and his family should receive.

Nurse's Aid
A specially trained individual who assists the nurse in caring for patients. Often involved in weighing, measuring, feeding, bathing, and comforting children.

Nurse practitioner
A nurse with advanced education who performs physical examinations, and engages in delivery of some care previously associated with physicians, such as the management of minor illnesses. Also, provides help in the management of daily problems.

Occupational Therapist
A specialist who helps with practical methods for overcoming disabilities. Encourages maximal functioning of arms and hands through adaptive equipment, exercises and short cuts derived from the experience of others. Particularly helpful in the areas of self-care and dressing.

Opthalmoscope
An instrument which doctors use to look inside the eye. Pressure from hydrocephalus or an ineffectively functioning shunt can sometimes be discovered this way.

Oral hygiene
Health care for the teeth and gums.

Orthopedist

A doctor who specializes in treatment (surgical and nonsurgical) of bones and joints.

Orthosis
A brace or similar device which strengthens or replaces bones, joints, or muscles in the body which do not work properly.

Orthotist
A specialist who designs and builds orthoses.

Ossify
When tissue (cartilage, muscle) turns to bone.

Osteotomy
Any operation in which a bone is cut into two parts. Usually the parts are put together again in a different way so as to correct a structural problem.

Parallel bars
Special bars that can be walked between. They enable the arms to be used for greater support and decrease the weight the legs must bear.

Parallel pusher
A type of parallel bars which is very light and can be moved along during walking.

Paralysis
Inability to move certain muscles, or to feel sensation (touch, temperature, pain). This can be complete or partial.

Paralympics
A special athletic competition for disabled competitors, operated in much the same way as the Olympics.

Paraplegia
Paralysis of the legs and lower part of the body.

Parapodium
A special device which helps paraplegic children stand upright at an early age. A type of orthosis.

Pediatrician
A physician who specializes in caring for children. Involved in curing some illnesses, preventing others, and managing problems related to chronic disabilities.

Pedigree
A detailed history of family ancestors.

Pedodontist
A dentist who specializes in the treatment of children.

Penile Appliance
A device that fits over the penis to collect urine.

Perceptual-motor disability
A type of learning problem where the brain does not correctly interpret messages which are seen or heard and translate them into motor activities. This makes it difficult to learn and appropriately react.

Phenolpthalein
A nonprescription medicine which stimulates bowel movements. It is present in Ex-lax®.

Physical therapist

A specialist who helps children improve their skills in ambulating and caring for themselves. Often involved in exercise programs to prevent contractures and in teaching children how to use their braces and special equipment.

Plantar flexion

Movement of the foot in the direction of the sole.

Plaque

The accumulation of food, bacteria and other matter around the teeth that leads to decay.

Polygenic

Many genes are involved in producing the characteristic rather than one.

Post-op, post-operative

The period following surgery.

Posterior

Situated behind or toward the back part as opposed to anterior.

Pneumoencephalogram, PEG

A special X-ray procedure where air is placed inside or around the brain so that it can be seen and evaluated.

Pneumonia

An infection in the lungs.

Prenatal detection

Any procedure which provides information about the infant while it is still in the uterus.

Prone

Lying on the abdomen.

Prosthesis

An artificial limb.

Prosthetist

A specialist who makes and fits artificial limbs.

Primary care

Care which deals with general problems, in this instance childhood ones. It includes immunizations and the care of such problems as colds and other childhhood illnesses. Ideally it is coordinated with specialty care when the child has spina bifida.

Psychologist

A specialist who evaluates and treats intellectual, emotional, or behavioral problems.

Pyelonephritis

An infection in one or both kidneys

Rectal prolapse

When part of the lower bowel extends through the anus and lies outside the body.

Rectum

The last portion of the large intestine ending at the anal canal.

Reduction of hips

Repositioning of the femur so that its upper end fits into the hip socket.

Regression
A return to a former or earlier state; going back; subsiding; such as when a child who is toilet trained temporarily loses this ability after a new baby arrives.

Reflux-urinary
When urine within the bladder moves backwards up the ureters toward the kidneys. Normally this does not occur.

Resident
A trained physician who is further specializing in some aspect of medicine, such as pediatrics, orthopedics, urology, etc.

RISA scan
A special procedure where radioactive material is placed into the cerebral spinal fluid. This is done through a lumbar puncture and the circulation of this fluid can then be observed.

Rounds
A general term which refers to doctors, nurses or other medical workers going around in a group to see or discuss the patients.

Sacral area
The area of the spine which lies between the buttocks and below the small of the back.

Scoliosis
A curvature of the spine toward the right or left side of the baby.

Scott device
A mechanical sphincter surgically placed in the male to control when the patient urinates. It is not currently available for wide patient use.

Senekot
A prescription medication to stimulate the movement of stool through the bowels.

Separation anxiety
Anxiety feelings or emotions experienced when separated from family and friends; feelings often mixed with fear and uncertainty.

Sexuality
A term which includes things that make a person feminine or masculine, e.g. attitudes, actions, self-image.

Sharrard procedure
An operation which helps keep the hip joint in its proper position.

Shunt
A shorthand term for any device which carries cerebrospinal fluid to another part of the body. Used when the normal pathways of cerebrospinal fluid circulation are obstructed.

Siblings
Brothers and sisters.

Social worker
A specialist skilled in counseling about emotional, social and financial stresses. There are many types of social workers functioning in a variety of ways.

Spastic

Muscles which are overly tense and difficult to control.

Specialty care

Care related primarily to a specific area. One area is that of children and families affected by spina bifida. Ideally it is coordinated with primary care.

Speech pathologist

A specialist who identifies the type and source of speech problems and provides a program of therapy to remedy it.

Spina bifida

The general term for the birth defect where the spinal column is not formed properly. There are many varieties of this defect and they vary in severity. (See myelomeningocele, meningocele, spina bifida occulta.)

Spica cast

A special cast which covers the lower trunk and upper legs. Used to keep the hip joint in the proper position.

Spinal fluid

The fluid which surrounds the brain and spinal cord. Also called cerebrospinal fluid.

Spinal fusion

An operation to join the spine bones so there is no movement between them.

Spinal tap

A procedure to remove some of the spinal fluid. A needle is placed into the fluid through the lower back or lumbar area. Also called a lumbar puncture.

Spinal column

The backbone composed of vertebrae and encasing the spinal cord.

Spinal cord

The nervous tissue which lies within the spinal column, and is connected to the brain.

Spina bifida occulta

A splitting or defect in the vertebrae which is hidden under the skin. The person usually has no symptoms.

Sphincters

The muscles surrounding the outlets from the bladder and rectum. They control the flow of urine and stool out of the body.

Stoma

An artificial opening to the outside of the body after diversionary surgery, usually the end of an ileal conduit in children with spina bifida.

Strabismus

When the eyes do not work together in looking at an object. They may turn inward or outward.

Stryker frame

A special bed which makes it easy to turn patients from front to back.

Stool

The body's waste products passed through the rectum (feces, bowel movements).

Supine
  Lying on the back.
Surgeon
  Any specialist who performs operations. There are many varieties such as neurosurgeon, orthopedist, urologist, and ophthalmologist.
Tendon transfer
  When a tendon from a muscle is moved to another position so the muscle will pull in a different direction.
Thoracic area
  The chest.
Thoracic spine
  The area of the spine which is in the chest.
Tofranil®
  A prescription medication which permits the bladder to store urine for a longer time.
Triple arthrodesis
  An operation on the foot which makes it more stable.
Turtle-like shells
  A body cast which supports the spine after surgery. It is made in two parts like a turtle's shell. The half in which the child is not resting can be removed.
Ultrasound
  A procedure where very rapid sound waves are directed into a pregnant mother's abdomen and their echos measured. This gives a picture of the unborn baby.
Ureter
  The tube which carries urine from the kidney to the bladder.
Urethra
  The tube which carries urine from the bladder to the outside of the body.
Urologist
  A surgical specialist who deals with the urinary system.
VA shunt, ventriculo-atrial shunt
  A shunt that passes from the ventricle in the brain to the atrium of the heart.
Varus
  Turned inward.
Valgus
  Turned outward.
Ventricle
  A space within the brain. There are four such spaces and most cerebrospinal fluid is produced in two of these and circulates between all four.
Ventriculitis
  An infection within the ventricles of the brain.
Ventriculogram
  An x-ray procedure where air is placed into the ventricles in the brain so their size and shape can be seen.

VP shunt, ventriculo-peritoneal shunt
   A shunt which runs from the ventricle of the brain to the abdominal cavity.
Vertebrae
   The bones which make up the spinal column.
Voiding cystourethrogram
   An x-ray procedure which shows the bladder and how urine is passed from the bladder to the outside of the body.
Walker
   A device which assists a disabled person to maintain balance while walking.
Well child care
   Another term for primary care.
Zymenol®
   A prescription chocolate-flavored mineral oil laxative.

INDEX

301